BUILDING A STRONG SENSE OF SELF

Embarking on the Journey of Change

THE INNER CONTROL *IS* THE TRUE CONTROL
Making Lasting Lifestyle and Behavioral Changes

BOOK 1

BUILDING A STRONG SENSE OF SELF

Embarking on the Journey of Change
Second Edition

A. Sehatti, RN, MSN
Family Nurse Practitioner

NCWC/Amend-Health Press

BUILDING A STRONG SENSE OF SELF: *Embarking on the Journey of Change* (1) **THE INNER CONTROL IS THE TRUE CONTROL:** *Making Lasting Lifestyle and Behavioral Changes.* **2nd Edition.** Copyright © 2022 by A. Sehatti, RN, MSN, Family Nurse Practitioner.

ISBN   978-0-578-34719-6   (paperback)

Addiction/Alcoholism   Eating Disorders   Weight Loss
Behavioral and Lifestyle Changes   Relationships   Building Self-Confidence
Personal Growth   Codependency   Emotional Health

Includes biographical references

The original work was published and copyrighted in May 2018 as THE INNER CONTROL IS THE TRUE CONTROL: *Making Lasting Lifestyle Changes* / BOOK 1-BUILDING A STRONG SENSE OF SELF

Printed and bounded in the United States of America
First Edition Copyrighted: May 2018; Revised Editions Copyrighted: August 2020, November 2021
Second Edition Copyrighted: January 2022; Revised Edition Copyrighted: November 2022

Published by:
NCWC/Amend-Health Press
AKA Nutritional Counseling and Weight Control Clinic
51 E. Campbell Avenue, Suite 129 - 154
Campbell, CA 95008
United States
www.NCWC-AmendHealthPress.com
www.EatActThinkHealthy.com

About the Author

A. Sehatti is a registered nurse and family nurse practitioner. She received her bachelor's degree in nursing from University of Pennsylvania and her master's degree in nursing from UCLA.

Aside from her clinical work at such places as Stanford, UCLA, and Caltech Health Center, she has over forty years of experience in educating adults and children on weight management, nutrition, and total wellness. The author currently works as a health educator and nutritional consultant at a private practice that she established in 2005 in Northern California.

A. Sehatti is highly dedicated to making a difference in people's lives. It has been the reward of witnessing people reach their health and wellness goals that has inspired her to write books and share the tools that have helped her clients with her readers.

Books Published by A. Sehatti

ACCOUNTABILITY AND EMPOWERMENT
A Four-Step Strategy for Overcoming Resentment
The Inner Control Is the True Control - Book 2

THE INNER CONTROL IS THE TRUE CONTROL
WORKBOOK, SECOND EDITION
Inspirational Scripts

A TOOL FOR LETTING GO OF RESENTMENT AND ANGER
Short. Straightforward. Transformative.

A WORKBOOK FOR OVERCOMING RESENTMENT
Mindfulness Scripts

A HANDBOOK FOR DEALING WITH SUGAR
CRAVINGS AND DEPENDENCY
NCWC's Nutrition 101 Series

NCWC'S NUTRITION 101 WORKBOOK
NCWC's Nutrition 101 Series

21-DAY LOG BOOK FOR ACHIEVING WELLNESS GOALS
NCWC's Nutrition 101 Series

A Heartfelt Thank You to:

My late husband, who inspired me to write books and helped me learn to trust my own judgments.

My daughter, my pride and joy, who has taught me to affirm myself. The most joyous moments of my life were those that I spent raising her.

My parents and sisters, who planted the seeds of compassion and resilience in me. In particular, my late father, whom I owe my love of reading and whose love made me work harder.

Andy and Shana, who took me in as one of their own during a critical period in my life. They had a significant impact in shaping who I am today.

All of my friends and relatives, who were there for me in my time of grief and beyond. Their support and kindness has made me believe even more in the miracle of human compassion.

Every single one of my clients, who have enriched my journey in a unique way. I sincerely appreciate their confidence in me.

*This book is dedicated to
my beloved late husband.*

The books in the series of *The Inner Control Is the True Control* were primarily written to help people reach their health goals (i.e., maintain weight loss or sobriety).

These works have achieved more than what they aimed for: In addition to helping people to make lasting lifestyle changes, they have empowered many couples to improve and transform their relationships.

A WORD OF CAUTION: Please be advised that *Building a Strong Sense of Self* delivers its message in a *forthright* manner.

This approach is used to help readers break down their wall of resistance (i.e., the defense mechanism of avoidance that protects our inner wounds in the short term but makes us remain stuck and face more emotional pain in the long term).

For this reason, some readers may experience a short-term inner turmoil as they work through some of the chapters in this book.

When the bandage that covers our inner wound
is removed and our vulnerable core is exposed,
we will naturally experience emotional pain.

It is when we allow ourselves to attend to our core wounds that we heal and become free to move onward and achieve our health goals—this may be why the books in the series of *The Inner Control Is the True Control* have been transformational for many people.

"Where you stumble, there lies your treasure."
—Joseph Campbell

"What you resist, persists."
—Carl Jung

"What you feel, you can heal."
—John Gray

Please note that this publication is not intended to replace the services offered by a mental health professional. When needed, the assistance of an expert in the area should be sought.

Contents

INTRODUCTION: CHANGING OUR MINDSET

How It All Started   3

The New Approach   6

About this Book   11

A Personal Note to My Readers   13

PART I: A DETERMINED, PROACTIVE, AND GOAL-ORIENTED MINDSET

CHAPTER 1   Perspective   19

CHAPTER 2   Motivational Inner Thoughts and Self-Talks   24

PART II: A FLEXIBLE, ADAPTABLE, AND TOLERANT MINDSET

CHAPTER 3   Perspective   31

CHAPTER 4   Validating and Affirming Inner Thoughts and Self-Talks   35

PART III: AN EMPOWERING AND CONSTRUCTIVE MINDSET

CHAPTER 5   Perspective   43

CHAPTER 6   Empowering Inner Thoughts and Self-Talks   54

CHAPTER 7   Constructive Communications and Behaviors   57

PART IV: A SUPPORTIVE, REALISTIC, AND LOGICAL MINDSET

CHAPTER 8   Perspective   65

CHAPTER 9   Nurturing Inner Thoughts and Self-Talks   81

PART V: A MINDFUL, CONSCIENTIOUS, AND EMPATHETIC MINDSET

CHAPTER 10   Perspective   89

CHAPTER 11   Emotional Healing: Empathy and Forgiveness   105

CHAPTER 12   Perceptive Inner Thoughts and Self-Talks   115

REFERENCES   121

INTRODUCTION

CHANGING OUR MINDSET

HOW IT ALL STARTED

After I lost my husband to cancer in 2005, I could no longer find a sense of purpose in working as a nurse practitioner. Now, I was not seeing patients in the exam room, I was seeing individuals in the real world. More than ever, I was thinking of the *total* person: the physical, emotional, and spiritual being.

Working as a nurse practitioner, I spent fifteen minutes with each patient. This short amount of time only allowed me to offer medical advice and prescribe medications when needed. In such a setting, I was only attending to the physical being while neglecting the rest—the emotional and spiritual needs of my patients. This was not rewarding or even acceptable to me anymore.

In that year, after much soul searching and deep contemplation, I quit working as a nurse practitioner and established my own practice, where I worked as a nutritionist and health educator and provided one-on-one health, nutritional, and weight management counseling for individuals with chronic health problems and weight issues.

In order to help my clients manage their weight and improve their total well-being, I focused on their diet, physical activity, and behavior.

Through providing in-depth health and nutritional education, I raised my clients' awareness and helped them to establish a healthy diet plan.

Daily cardio workout routines that were tailored to their own specific health conditions, interests, and schedules were implemented. Strength training workouts were encouraged to increase bone density, lean muscle mass, and metabolism.

In the area of behavioral modification, general stress management techniques and impulse control strategies were discussed and reinforced throughout the follow-up visits. Helpful behavioral tips for healthy eating while eating out or during the holidays and social occasions were provided.

This traditional approach led to significant weight loss and remarkable improvement in the health condition of my clients as was acknowledged by their primary care providers. However, a few years into the practice, I felt compelled to pause and reevaluate this method as many of my clients regressed to their old ways and gradually regained the weight they had lost. With this in mind, I spent an extensive amount of time making observations, reflecting, studying human behavior, and searching for answers.

The hard and long work redirected my attention towards the behavior modification aspect of my practice and impelled me to explore this area more deeply and extensively. Thus, I examined the traditional and contemporary school of thoughts in western psychology, such as family therapy, positive psychology, cognitive behavioral therapy, and psychodynamic psychotherapy.

I investigated the latest findings in the field of neurobiology of the brain and delved into brain plasticity. I explored the ancient wisdom of eastern philosophies such as Buddhism and contemplated at length on such concepts as mindfulness, empathy, and self-compassion.

Ultimately, it was through the deep sense of connection that I had developed with my clients, in addition to the knowledge that I had gained on my own journey of growth, that I was able to find the answer that I was looking for: people's conditioned patterns of thoughts during the stressful times impacted their feelings and drove their automatic stress responses (i.e., binge eating or drinking).

In other words, people's emotional experiences gradually led them to return to their old habits and regain the weight they had lost. This premise served as the foundation for the new and more effective approach in helping my clients achieve lasting lifestyle changes and maintain their weight loss.

THE NEW APPROACH

While I continued to encourage healthy eating and regular physical activity, under the new approach, I placed more emphasis on behavior modification—particularly, during times of stress.

Realizing that as humans, we have little control over stressors that create challenging experiences in our lives, I turned my focus to another area where we have more control: our internal dialogues that drive our responses to the stressor—our state of mind or *mindset*.

Based on the belief that we have more control over our state of mind, I arrived at the following reasoning: A fundamental change in our mindset changes the way we perceive our own image, the world around us, and the experiences we have. In turn, these perceptions directly impact the way we act, respond, and take care of ourselves.

Therefore, I concluded that focusing on my clients' patterns of conscious and unconscious inner thoughts and self-talks may be the key to helping them reach lasting behavioral and lifestyle changes. This conclusion was reached based on the following observations and premises (Figure 1 on Page 8):

> » When we are on autopilot, our past experiences may, subconsciously, impact the way we view and interpret a present situation.

» This perception, which may or may not accurately represent the current event, becomes *our reality*. For example, during a difficult situation, an unresolved issue from our childhood that was buried deep in our subconscious may resurface and negatively impact our perception of what is happening in the present. This distorted perception becomes our reality— what we may falsely refer to as the fact.

» When a *distorted reality* is left unchecked, it triggers dysfunctional thoughts and internal dialogues. In turn, this distorted mindset generates negative feelings (e.g., shame).

» As we have remained unawakened, these painful feelings trigger a set of automatic responses that were programmed in us during our childhood (e.g., blaming others when we are faced with our own wrongdoings). These behaviors, which protected and insulated us as children, become maladaptive later in life as they lead to negative outcomes (e.g., people's angry and retaliatory reactions) and emotional pain.

» When our inner turmoil is left unresolved, we may seek comfort in food, alcohol, or other substances/activities in order to regain a sense of inner peace and normalcy.

» Repeating such patterns of mindless and maladaptive behaviors results in unintended negative consequences such as poor lifestyle choices, dependencies/addictions, weight issues, suboptimal physical and/or mental health, dysfunctional relationships, financial instability, and a poor quality of life.

❦ ❦ ❦

As a result of implementing the new strategy, my clients gained insight into themselves and became more aware of their hidden thoughts, self-talks, and defense mechanisms.

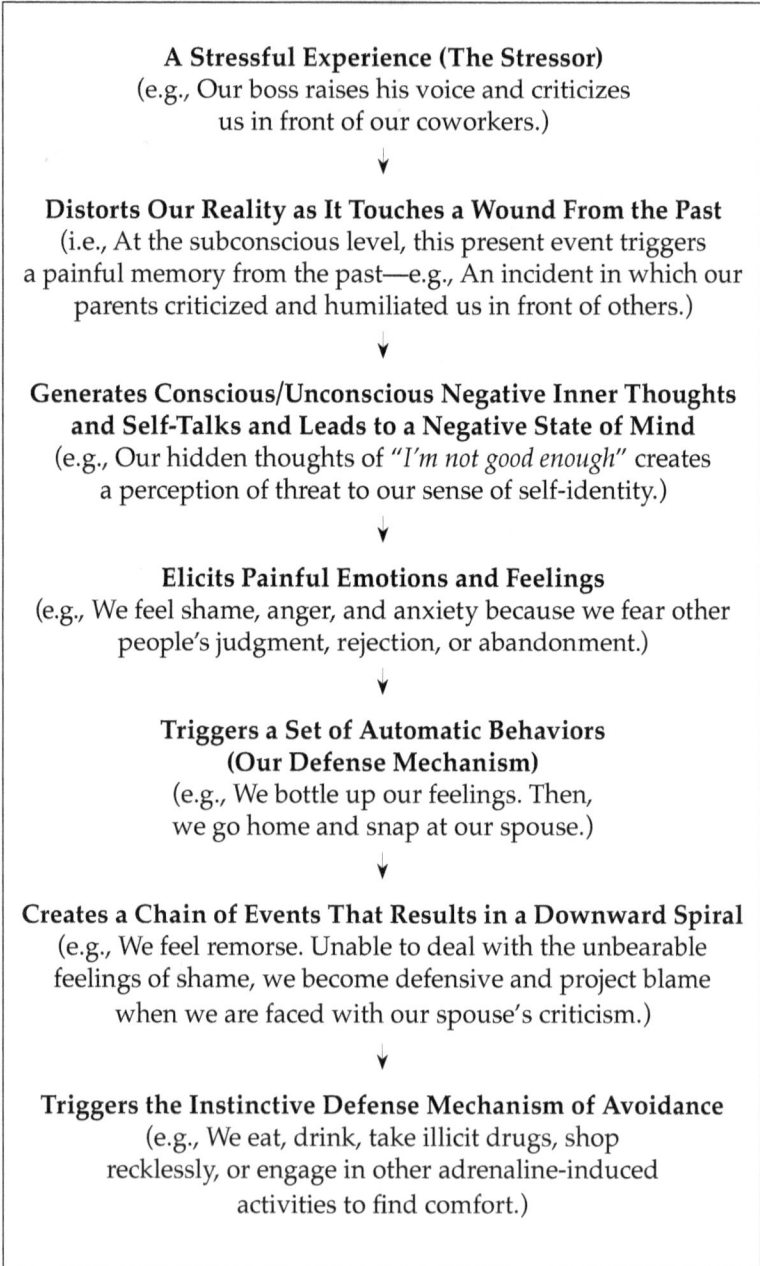

Figure 1

A Stressful Experience (The Stressor)
(e.g., Our boss raises his voice and criticizes
us in front of our coworkers.)

↓

Distorts Our Reality as It Touches a Wound From the Past
(i.e., At the subconscious level, this present event triggers
a painful memory from the past—e.g., An incident in which our
parents criticized and humiliated us in front of others.)

↓

**Generates Conscious/Unconscious Negative Inner Thoughts
and Self-Talks and Leads to a Negative State of Mind**
(e.g., Our hidden thoughts of *"I'm not good enough"* creates
a perception of threat to our sense of self-identity.)

↓

Elicits Painful Emotions and Feelings
(e.g., We feel shame, anger, and anxiety because we fear other
people's judgment, rejection, or abandonment.)

↓

**Triggers a Set of Automatic Behaviors
(Our Defense Mechanism)**
(e.g., We bottle up our feelings. Then,
we go home and snap at our spouse.)

↓

Creates a Chain of Events That Results in a Downward Spiral
(e.g., We feel remorse. Unable to deal with the unbearable
feelings of shame, we become defensive and project blame
when we are faced with our spouse's criticism.)

↓

Triggers the Instinctive Defense Mechanism of Avoidance
(e.g., We eat, drink, take illicit drugs, shop
recklessly, or engage in other adrenaline-induced
activities to find comfort.)

Since they were no longer living on autopilot, they were able to see their own imperfections—their humanness. By taking responsibility for their own parts in their emotional suffering, they became empowered to see choices, heal through forgiveness, and form a new set of principles that governed a more positive mindset. This positive outlook fostered a sense of compassion, empathy, and acceptance towards themselves and others; produced actions that supported self-care; and generated a sense of empowerment that helped them to effectively resolve issues during difficult times.

Not being enslaved to their old habits, my clients felt liberated and empowered to make better choices and achieve their weight loss and other health-related goals.

Going through this long and difficult path, my clients came to view relapses as a natural part of the process of change and as an opportunity for further learning and growth: each time they regressed to their old habits, they learned to take a few steps back, reflect, and gain insight; learn from their mistakes; change their negative self-thoughts; forgive; and commit to new ways of thinking.

In addition to weight loss, lasting behavioral and lifestyle changes, and improved physical and mental health, the new approach resulted in many other remarkable positive outcomes in the lives of my clients: better personal and work relationships, a higher self-esteem, and a more positive self-image.

In sum, people who went through the process of change and transformation experienced remarkable positive changes in the way they viewed and perceived themselves, others, and their life experiences. Through gaining *control over their ways of thinking*, they learned to control their actions and behaviors. No longer behaving automatically, they were able to make better choices and feel more in *control of their own lives*.

Control Over Our Inner Thoughts →	Control Over Our Behaviors →	Control Over Our Lives
INNER CONTROL	TRUE CONTROL	TOTAL WELLNESS

✿ ✿ ✿

In conclusion, witnessing my clients achieve their weight loss goals and sustain their transformational changes has convinced me that lasting behavioral and lifestyle changes are attainable—in particular, when we are ready to face the harsh truths (i.e., our imperfections and/or those of our loved ones).

Furthermore, observing the positive outcomes in my clients' lives has reinforced the belief that gaining control over our mindset empowers us to have control over our emotional experiences, the choices we make, the people we decide to surround ourselves with, and the lifestyle we choose to have. It may then be plausible to conclude that the fundamental change in our ways of thinking is the key to reaching total wellness.

As the years have gone by, I have gained more experience and understanding in helping people meet their physical, emotional, and spiritual needs and reach their targets. In pursuing a greater purpose and in response to my clients' encouragements and insistence, I will be sharing my approach in attaining lasting lifestyle changes with my readers through a series of three books. It is my utmost hope that reading these books would also inspire you to maximize your potential for living a healthy and fulfilled life.

> *The Inner Control Is the True Control:*
> *Gaining control over our thoughts and self-talks*
> *will empower us to gain control over our behaviors*
> *and sustain our healthy lifestyle changes.*

ABOUT THIS BOOK

By inspiring you to cultivate principles and values that foster positive self-talks, *Building a Strong Sense of Self* helps you stick to your healthy behavioral changes and achieve your health goals:

A positive mindset generates
self-compassion, -accountability, -forgiveness, and -empowerment;

Drives constructive behaviors and enables us to stay in
control and make better choices; and,

Empowers us to stay resilient;
maintain our self-care practices in the face of setbacks
and times of stress; and, reach total wellness.

Part I through Part V in this book explore and promote the following positive mindsets, respectively: determined, proactive, and goal-oriented; flexible, adaptable, and tolerant; empowering and constructive; supportive, realistic, and logical; and, mindful, conscientious, and empathetic.

All of the five parts start with a perspective—viewpoints that are intended to raise awareness and trigger critical thinking. These thought-provoking concepts also serve as a foundation for a set of related inner thoughts and self-talks that is presented at the end of each section.

Although every effort has been made to present the materials in a way that would facilitate easy reading, brief pauses are highly recommended for greater absorption as well as for regaining a sense of inner peace.

The outlining format and self-dialogues (at the end of each section) are designed to slow down one's reading. This strategy is used to increase concentration, raise attention, and stimulate further thinking.

Please note that the companion to this book, *The Inner Control Is the True Control Workbook,* offers inspirational scripts that are crafted in such a way to directly correspond to each part of this book. Reading these scripts at the end of each corresponding section will reinforce learning and help you gain a sense of inner calmness.

A PERSONAL NOTE TO
MY READERS

While reading *Building a Strong Sense of Self*, please keep in mind that this book was written based on the following premises and personal philosophies:

1. A true transformation and personal growth may not be attained unless we examine the past and make sense of what happened during the early years of our childhood.

2. This book delivers academic and clinical knowledge as well as insights that were gained through personal observations straightforwardly, candidly, and in a forthright manner due to the following beliefs:

   a. As mature adults, we are all capable of facing the truth.

   b. Insincere communication (i.e., withholding, sugar-coating, or distorting the truth) not only is unhelpful and disrespectful but also may be damaging.

   c. Judging and labeling ourselves is harmful—it limits our potential for personal growth. In contrast, making non-judgmental observations and labeling our *behaviors* as experienced by others (e.g., *controlling, aggressive, or victimizing*) can be transformative—it may help us understand how our behaviors make other people feel and contribute to our emotional suffering.

   d. It is only when we are willing to face our truth that we

get a chance to better ourselves, improve our lives in a meaningful way, and reach the lasting happiness that we deserve to experience.

3. This book defines the term "awakened" as:

    A state-of-being in which we are aware of our inner thoughts, feelings, and behaviors. This state of awareness helps us become mindful, make sense of our experience, and see the truth.

    When we are mindful, we build a deeper connection with other people since we can better understand their thoughts, feelings, and behaviors and relate to their experiences.

    Our mindful and understanding mindset allows us to observe ourselves and others in a non-judgmental manner.

4. *Building a Strong Sense of Self* provokes introspection and raises awareness. Thus, some painful truths or memories from the past may naturally resurface to the level of conscious awareness and generate inner turmoil. For this reason, please read this book with an open mind and forgiving heart towards yourself and those who may have failed you. Re-reading the inspirational scripts in *The Inner Control Is the True Control Workbook* is highly recommended for reaching a state of inner calmness.

PART I

**A DETERMINED, PROACTIVE,
AND GOAL-ORIENTED MINDSET**

To make 'lasting' behavioral and lifestyle changes, we first become aware of our unhelpful thinking patterns that drive our unhealthy habits; then, we develop and cultivate a more constructive set of inner thoughts and self-talks that empowers us to gain control and make better choices.

In other words, to be able to maintain our behavioral changes and achieve our health goals, we may need to make a fundamental change in 'the way we think'.

A constructive and positive outlook that is executed by the prefrontal cortex part of our brain keeps our instinctive impulses in check and helps us stay in control and sustain our healthy lifestyle changes.

Working through the journey of change can be an uphill battle: Even when we work diligently through the process, we may still encounter challenges and revert back to our old habits.

However, when we are 'determined' to achieve our goals, make great 'efforts' to overcome challenges (i.e., temptations), and 'persevere' in the face of setbacks, then we become empowered to learn from our mistakes, commit to new ways of thinking and behaving, and move onward.

1

PERSPECTIVE

The viewpoints presented in this chapter will serve as the foundation for the motivational internal thoughts and self-talks that are outlined in Chapter 2.

※ ※ ※

To adopt and *maintain* behavioral and lifestyle changes, we may need to: 1) Focus on the present moment and grow mindful; 2) Become aware of our unhelpful thinking patterns that drive our unhealthy behaviors; and, 3) Develop and cultivate a mindset that empowers us to gain control and make better choices.

Working through this process can become an uphill battle: Even when we work diligently through the steps, we may still encounter challenges, come to a *pause,* and revert back to our old habits (although we learn that these pauses or regressions are a natural part of the process of change and *can* be overcome—we *can* get our life back on the right path again when we go back and retake those steps).

However, there may be times that we come to a *halt*: we regress to our old patterns of thinking and behaving but we are unable to regain our control and get our life back on the right path again. Feeling frustrated, exhausted, and *stuck*, we give up and gradually return to living on autopilot and in a mechanical manner. Why is that? Why do we come to a 'halt' and become stuck on our journey of change? The following section may provoke introspection and help provide some answers.

※ ※ ※

It has been theorized that humans *instinctively seek pleasure* (i.e., we like to receive affirmation, approval, praise, and reward) and *avoid displeasure* (i.e., we don't like to receive negative feedback, face our mistakes, or deal with setbacks).

As mentioned earlier, discovering our faulty ways of thinking, which drive our unhealthy habits (i.e., our flawed character-traits), is an essential step in the process of *true* change. However, discovering our flaws is not a pleasant experience; it can generate such painful emotions as shame, guilt, and anxiety.

Consequently, the journey of transformation could produce inner turmoil (i.e., displeasure) and become a painful and difficult task to undertake. However, when we *face* our flaws and *cope* with our inner turmoil, then we become empowered to hold ourselves accountable, see choices, make changes, learn from our mistakes, and move onward on our journey of change.

On the other hand, when we use defense mechanisms (i.e., avoidance) to stop our inner turmoil, then we may not face our flaws and be able to make constructive changes. As a result, we will continue to experience setbacks over and over again. Feeling stressed and stuck, we may eventually give up on our journey.

The following scenarios may help us see how using defense mechanisms to avoid experiencing displeasure could eventually hamper our personal growth and make us feel stuck on our journey of change.

Scenario 1: When we learn about our flaws and experience inner turmoil, we project or redirect our negative emotions in order to find relief. For example,

> » We blame people in our past (i.e., our parents) for our faulty habits and weaknesses;
>
> » We become resentful towards those individuals who pointed out our mistakes or helped us see our flaws; or,

» We focus on the flaws of others (i.e., we analyze and fix people in our immediate environment).

In such situations, we inadvertently add to our emotional pain. Feeling emotionally drained, exhausted, and stuck, we give up on our journey.

Scenario 2: When we learn about our mistakes and experience inner turmoil, we seek comfort in food, alcohol, or other substances. Afterwards, we become remorseful and experience anticipatory anxiety (i.e., fear of failure that is evoked by the memory of past failed attempts to reach our goal). Feeling discouraged and stuck, we give up.

Scenario 3: When we learn about our flaws, instead of changing our mindset, we change our behaviors and develop a *functioning self* (a self-defense maneuver to shield ourselves against others' judgment, rejection, or abandonment). This *pseudo self* stops us from staying true to ourselves, facing and resolving issues, and moving onward on our journey.

Sometimes, even after building emotional resilience, we may still face setbacks and feel stuck on our journey of change.

Why is that?

Could this have to do with our environment (e.g., people in our social circle, our significant other, family, friends, or social media)?

For example, is it possible that we feel stuck and revert back to our old habits because, while we are changing, people in our immediate environment are not (since they are not going through the journey with us)?

The following scenarios may help us see how such a situation could stop our personal growth and make us feel stuck on our journey of change.

Scenario 4: People who generally tend to over-identify with us and over-empathize with our feelings may inadvertently persuade us (*enable us*) to give up when we experience inner turmoil and stumble on our journey.

Scenario 5: Feeling threatened by our personal growth, those who tend to over function for us to gain a sense of inner normalcy undermine our efforts and inadvertently hamper our growth.

Scenario 6: We face challenges when we perceive that our friends are feeling intimidated by our transformation. Fearing their rejection, judgment, or abandonment, we gradually regress to our old ways and feel stuck.

Scenario 7: We experience self-doubt and feel stuck on our journey when we remain in unhealthy relationships with people who resist change and continue to engage in avoidance defense mechanisms.

Scenario 8: We struggle to sustain our healthy behavioral changes when our faulty habits are *enabled* by those in our immediate environment who are unable to hold us accountable in a firm, consistent, and healthy manner. Unable to make progress, we feel frustrated and stuck.

Scenario 9: We are unable to sustain our behavioral changes because our faulty habits are *reinforced* by people who share the same character traits. Being frustrated by our lack of progress, we feel stuck.

In conclusion, to prevail on the journey of change, we need to build emotional resilience, become proactive, and set ourselves for success (i.e., create a healthy environment that would support personal growth and change).

🌊 🌊 🌊

In sum, to achieve lasting behavioral and lifestyle changes, we have to make a fundamental change in *the way we think.*

A constructive outlook that is executed by our prefrontal cortex keeps our instinctive impulses in check and drives healthy behaviors. In other words, our new ways of thinking empowers us to take control, make better choices, and *sustain* our healthy behavioral and lifestyle changes.

Working through the process of change can be an uphill battle; it requires *determination, great efforts,* and *perseverance.*

Relapses or regressions to our old ways are a natural part of the process of change. When we are *determined* to reach our goals, make *great efforts* to overcome challenges (i.e., our impulses and temptations), and continue to *persevere* in the face of setbacks, then we come to view *pauses* and *halts* as opportunities for further learning and growth: Each time that we regress to our old habits, we hold ourselves accountable in a non-judgmental manner, learn from our mistakes, commit to new ways of thinking and behaving, and move onward.

> *Making lasting* behavioral and lifestyle changes requires *determination, great efforts,* and *perseverance.*

2

MOTIVATIONAL INNER THOUGHTS AND SELF-TALKS

This chapter lists a set of motivational internal thoughts and dialogues that are driven by *a determined, proactive, and goal-oriented mindset* (i.e., a mindset that is gained through the process of personal growth and transformation).

❧ ❧ ❧

» In order to achieve lasting behavioral and lifestyle changes and reach total wellness, I will *build emotional resilience.*

- ○ I will believe in myself; I will not allow my mistakes or flaws to define me: I will separate my faulty ways of thinking and behaving (my flaws) from my *Self* (*The Person Within*).

- ○ I will cherish my strengths and take pride in my accomplishments; I will *support* myself in turning my weaknesses into my strengths.

» I will *set myself up for success*: I will make realistic goals and create a healthy environment that would support personal growth.

- ○ I will believe in other people; I will not define others by their flawed character-traits: I will separate their faulty ways of thinking and behaving from *The Person Within* (their *self*).

- ○ I will not fix people; Rather, I will focus on my own flaws and shape my environment as I lead by example.

- ○ Instead of reverting back to my old maladaptive ways, I will support and empower others in my environment to transform and meet me on the continuum of personal growth.

- ◦ I will become enlightened by gaining insight and enlighten others by expressing myself.

- ◦ Through setting and maintaining my healthy boundaries, I will remain strong and separate and take equal posturing in my relationships.

- ◦ My journey with others is effecting change together: When I change, others will change; When others change, I will change.

» Although the journey of change is challenging, I will go through this life-changing process because I deserve to live a fulfilled life.

Our journey with others is effecting change together: When we change, others will change; When others change, we will change.

PART II

**A FLEXIBLE, ADAPTABLE,
AND TOLERANT MINDSET**

While I cherish my strengths and take pride in my accomplishments, I realize that my advantages, greatness, gifts, talents, or skills do not define me or make me superior.

While I support myself in turning my weaknesses into my strengths, I realize that my imperfections, flaws, or limitations do not define me or make me inferior.

3

PERSPECTIVE

The following concepts will serve as the foundation for the validating and affirming inner thoughts and self-talks that are presented in Chapter 4.

🦚 🦚 🦚

We are born with a set of innate physical, mental, and emotional traits that are unique and specific to each one of us. Since we are *born* with these characteristics, they are ingrained in us; therefore, we cannot change them. Some examples of innate characteristics are one's gender and skin pigmentation.

These inherent traits are neither good nor bad; they make us neither superior nor inferior. They only represent our uniqueness.

In contrast to our innate characteristics, we are not born with our character traits (Figure 2). These characteristics are subjective constructs that consist of our predominant patterns of thinking (i.e., our core values, attitudes, and how we view our world), feeling (i.e., how we feel our emotions), and behaving (i.e., the way we express our thoughts and feelings). Therefore, our character traits (our attitudes, feelings, and behaviors) are neither unique nor specific to us.

These character traits are mainly developed during the early years of our childhood as we interact with our immediate environment. Although many factors such as our birth order, siblings, friends, schooling, society, religion, and culture play important roles in shaping our attitudes and behaviors, many psychologists believe that our parents or parent figures, who generally constitute our immediate environment, have the most impact on our character trait formation.

Figure 2

Innate Traits and Character Traits

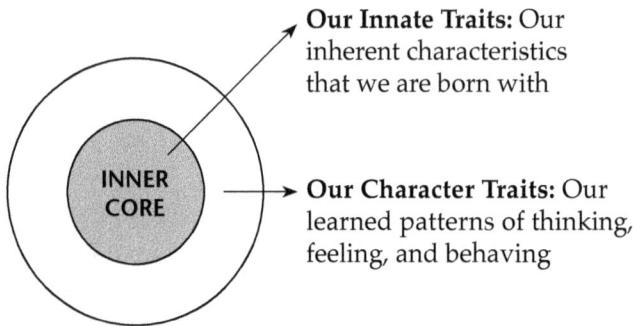

Our Innate Traits: Our inherent characteristics that we are born with

Our Character Traits: Our learned patterns of thinking, feeling, and behaving

INNER CORE

Our ways of thinking, feeling, and behaving that we learn in the early years become conditioned in us when our parents enable us to practice them through such parenting behaviors as rewarding (e.g., praising) or neglecting (e.g., being disengaged).

These conditioned attitudes and behaviors are later reinforced by the environment we live in (e.g., school, social media, church, and society) as we transition into adulthood.

When we remain unaware as adults, these learned and conditioned character-traits become automatic and part of our personality as though they were ingrained in us. This may explain why many of our patterns of thoughts, feelings, and behaviors are hidden from our conscious awareness when we live on autopilot.

🙨 🙨 🙨

Our character traits become fully formed and conditioned in us well before we reach the age of eighteen.

Since we are *not* born with these traits, we *can* change them: We *can* change the way we think, feel, and behave.

However, when we remain unaware and live our life on autopilot, we lose the opportunity to reevaluate our behaviors and discover our flawed ways of thinking that lead to our maladaptive coping responses.

In such situations, we will continue to mindlessly respond (think, feel, and behave) to our environment based on a set of misguided beliefs that are not constructive to reaching our full potential.

Therefore, when we remain unawakened, it may be impossible for us to fundamentally change our character traits—we may learn new skills (e.g., anger management) but we may not be able to experience a true lasting transformation.

🖜 🖜 🖜

As discussed earlier, our character traits are not fixed entities in us. In fact, human development is a continual process that happens over our lifetime—it starts at birth and ends when we die. As long as we live and interact with our environment (i.e., people), we act upon it, respond to it, and change it. Accordingly, we become transformed by the way it responds to us. Therefore, we are continually changing and developing (even when we remain unawakened).

In short, through our own actions and interactions with our environment, we will transform. As we change, our environment (i.e., people whom we interact with) will change.

Perhaps then, we could come to this conclusion: if we are not fixed entities, then we are always in a state of *being*. For this reason, *labeling, defining, or identifying ourselves merely based upon our character traits may be unfair and even damaging* as it could limit our growth and lead to negative emotional experiences.

4

VALIDATING AND AFFIRMING
INNER THOUGHTS AND SELF-TALKS

This chapter lists a set of validating and affirming internal thoughts and dialogues that are driven by *a flexible, adaptable, and tolerant mindset* (i.e., a mindset that is gained through the process of personal growth and transformation).

🌊 🌊 🌊

» I affirm and acknowledge my *total self*:

- ○ I acknowledge my innate traits:

    > Realizing that I was born with my unique set of inherited characteristics allows me to see my *uniqueness* and *individuality*. Therefore, I will appreciate myself as I am; *I am unique.*

- ○ I acknowledge my character traits—my ways of thinking, feeling, and behaving:

    > Being aware of my own thoughts and feelings stops me from neglecting my needs or dismissing my realities. Being mindful of my behaviors enables me to embrace my strengths and support myself in improving my weaknesses.

» Realizing that I developed my character traits during my childhood:

- ○ Stops me from judging myself by my flawed ways of thinking, feeling, and behaving.

- Helps me recognize that my imperfections and mistakes do not define my inner core (*Me*).

- Empowers me because I no longer see myself trapped: I always have a choice; If I *choose* to, I *can* change my ways of *being* (thinking, feeling, and behaving).

> *Our positive mindset helps us see a true image of our 'self':*
>
> *We don't have to be perfect, superior, or special to be adequate.*
>
> *We are unique; We are adequate.*

❧ ❧ ❧

The insight that I have gained into myself empowers me to better understand and relate to other individuals. Now, I can extend my positive mindset towards others:

» I affirm and acknowledge others' *total self*:

- I acknowledge other people's innate traits:

    Recognizing that others were born with their unique set of inherent characteristics allows me to see their *uniqueness* and individuality. Therefore, I will acknowledge people as *they* are. Now, I think of us all as *equals; I am neither inferior nor superior to anyone.*

- I recognize and accept people's character traits—their ways of thinking, feeling, and behaving:

    This awareness stops me from dismissing or neglecting the realities, opinions, desires, or feelings of others.

» Acknowledging that people learned their character traits during the early years of their childhood helps me realize that their mistakes or flawed ways of thinking, feeling, and behaving do not define *them*. This awareness:

- Empowers me to understand and relate to other people's experiences, instead of judging or labeling *them*.

- Offers me hope: when I regard and treat everyone with kindness, respect, and dignity, then I may be able to modify and transform the way people respond to me. *As I gain more rewarding experiences, I change and develop more compassion, tolerance, and patience towards myself and others.*

Our positive outlook enables us to see a true image of other people:

Others don't have to be perfect, superior, or special to be adequate.

Every person is unique; Everyone is adequate.

🐚 🐚 🐚

When I focus on my own *self*,
I am not being self-absorbed.

When I make a healthy environment for myself,
I am not being antisocial.

When I engage in self-care,
I am not being selfish.

When I stop sacrificing my physical, mental, or
emotional needs to attend to those of others,
I am not being egocentric.

So, without being enabling,
I will be kind and understanding to *the child in me;*
It is only then that I can be the best I could ever be.

When I am the best that I could ever be,
then I can be patient, tolerant, and understanding.

When I am the best that I could ever be,
then I can genuinely care for other people.

When I am the best that I could ever be,
then I can give without expecting anything in return.

When I am the best that I could ever be,
then I can see that others matter, too.

So, I Matter!

PART III

AN EMPOWERING AND
CONSTRUCTIVE MINDSET

"Too late he [Sir Thomas] became aware how unfavorable to the character of any young people, must be the totally opposite treatment which Maria and Julia had been always experiencing at home, where the excessive indulgence and flatter of their aunt had been continually contrasted with his own severity. He saw how ill he had judged, in expecting to counteract what was wrong in Mrs. Norris, by its reverse in himself, clearly saw that he had but increased the evil, by teaching them to repress their spirits in his presence, as to make their real disposition unknown to him, and sending them for all their indulgences to a person who had been able to attach them only by the blindness of her affection, and the excess of her praise.

Here had been grievous mismanagement; but bad as it was, he gradually grew to feel that it had not been the most direful mistake in his plan of education. Something must have been wanting within, or time would have worn away much of its ill effect. He feared that principle, active principle, had been wanting, that they had never been properly taught to govern their inclinations and tempers, by that sense of duty which can alone suffice. They had been instructed theoretically in their religion, but never required to bring it into daily practice. To be distinguished for elegance and accomplishments—the authorised [authorized] object of their youth—could have had no useful influence that way, no moral effect on the mind. He had meant them be good, but his cares had been directed to the understanding and manners, not the disposition; and of the necessity of self-denial and humility, he feared they had never heard from any lips that could profit them."

Jane Austin, Mansfield Park (London, England: Penguin Classics, Revised edition 2003), Volume III Chapter XVII, Page 430

5

PERSPECTIVE

The following concepts will serve as the foundation for the empowering internal thoughts and self-talks and constructive communications and behaviors that are outlined in Chapters 6 and 7, respectively.

🦅° 🦅° 🦅°

As natural and healthy children, we are born with certain primitive characteristics such as the reflex of sucking (i.e., a newborn automatically begins to suck right after birth). These natural characteristics of healthy children are mainly controlled by the primitive part of our brain. Naturally, our primitive mind generates emotions, internal thoughts, and behaviors that are instinctive, automatic, impulsive, self-centered, responsive, and reactive.

Figure 3 on Page 44 briefly outlines the state of mind (i.e., desires, needs, and ways of thinking) of a natural and healthy child.

Figure 3

The Inherent Mindset of Natural
and Healthy Children

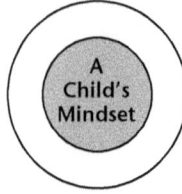

A Child's Mindset

I matter;
No one else matters!
I'm important;
No one is as important as me!

I'm special;
No one is as special as me!
My needs matter;
No one's needs are greater than mine!

I have to get what I want, the way
I want it, and when I want it!

*I want what I want **NOW**!*
I'm only interested in instant gratification;
I don't care what happens later.

I only want to play, have fun, and experience
***pleasure**.*

I experience pleasure when:
- I get what I want.
- I receive attention, approval,
praise, or reward.
- I'm right.
- I win; and,
You cheer for me.

Figure 3

The Inherent Mindset of Natural and
Healthy Children (Cont'd)

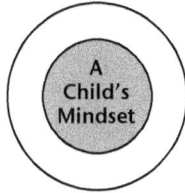

A
Child's
Mindset

*When I experience pleasure, I feel
safe, loved, and protected.
When I feel safe and secure, then I will smile at
you and love you (because I feel happy).*

*I don't like to feel **displeasure.***

*I experience displeasure when:
- I'm neglected.
- I can't get what I want.
- I'm held accountable.
- I'm controlled or kept from doing
what I want to do.
- I'm frowned at or shouted at.
- I'm punished.*

*These unpleasant experiences make me feel
unloved and insecure—like I'm not good enough.*

*When I feel unloved and insecure:
- I will not like you.
- I will cry and throw a tantrum to punish you.
- I will cry and throw a tantrum to
control you (so that I get what I want).*

*When I get what I want, then
I will be happy again; Then, I will like you.*

Figure 3

The Inherent Mindset of Natural and
Healthy Children (Cont'd)

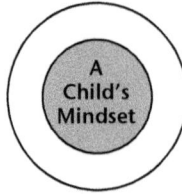

A
Child's
Mindset

I'm defenseless and helpless:
I need to be defended, protected,
and taken care of.

I'm fragile:
*I need to **avoid displeasure**.*
Therefore, I will do anything to
***avoid punishment**.*

I'm special:
*I need to experience **pleasure**.*
Therefore, I will please you and do
all of those things that would
***bring rewards**.*

When, as healthy children, we interact with a less than ideal environment, then we may become exposed to stressful experiences that generate painful emotions in us (e.g., guilt, shame, and anger).

Unable to learn healthy coping strategies from our unsuitable environment, we resort to the primitive and instinctive defense mechanism of aggression to express ourselves and gain a sense of inner security in times of stress.

When the display of overt aggression becomes discouraged or punished by our immediate environment—without it being replaced by a healthy coping strategy—then, we learn to use the defense mechanism (i.e., covert-aggression or passivity) that is modeled by one or both of our parents (or parent figures) in order to cope with our painful emotions.

The *unresolved* negative emotions and experiences of the early years of our childhood may become repressed and stored in the area of the brain that governs emotion and memory (the limbic system).

When we remain unawakened as adults, a stimulus (i.e., a similar experience) may easily trigger the neurons in this region and evoke the painful emotions that our brain remembers.

At the subconscious level, these triggered sensations may distort our perception of the present reality and bring about negative inner thoughts and feelings.

Being on autopilot, we may automatically respond to our painful emotions and feelings by using the same conditioned defense mechanism (i.e., overt-aggression, covert-aggression, or passivity) that we used as a child to cope with our inner unrest (Figure 4).

Figure 5 on Page 49 illustrates how a conditioned pathway in our brain leads to relapses and an unhealthy lifestyle when we suffer from a distorted self-image—an image that was primarily formed in us in the early years of our childhood.

Figure 4

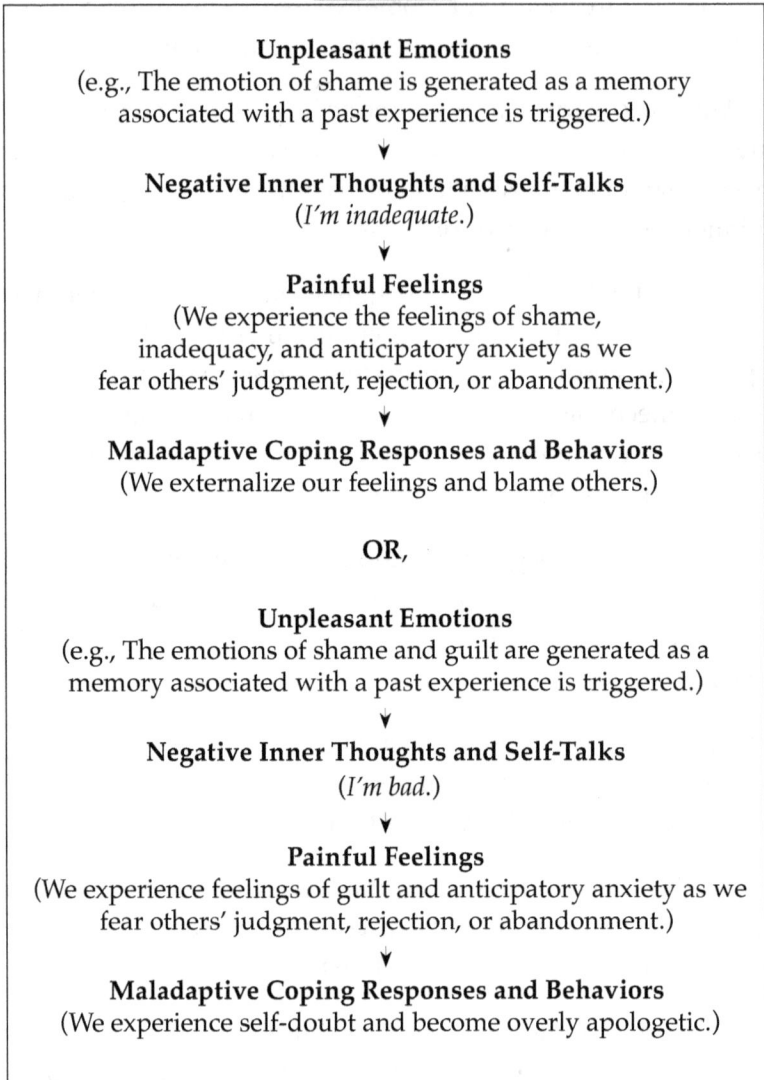

Unpleasant Emotions
(e.g., The emotion of shame is generated as a memory
associated with a past experience is triggered.)

Negative Inner Thoughts and Self-Talks
(*I'm inadequate.*)

Painful Feelings
(We experience the feelings of shame,
inadequacy, and anticipatory anxiety as we
fear others' judgment, rejection, or abandonment.)

Maladaptive Coping Responses and Behaviors
(We externalize our feelings and blame others.)

OR,

Unpleasant Emotions
(e.g., The emotions of shame and guilt are generated as a
memory associated with a past experience is triggered.)

Negative Inner Thoughts and Self-Talks
(*I'm bad.*)

Painful Feelings
(We experience feelings of guilt and anticipatory anxiety as we
fear others' judgment, rejection, or abandonment.)

Maladaptive Coping Responses and Behaviors
(We experience self-doubt and become overly apologetic.)

Figure 5

The Relapse Process

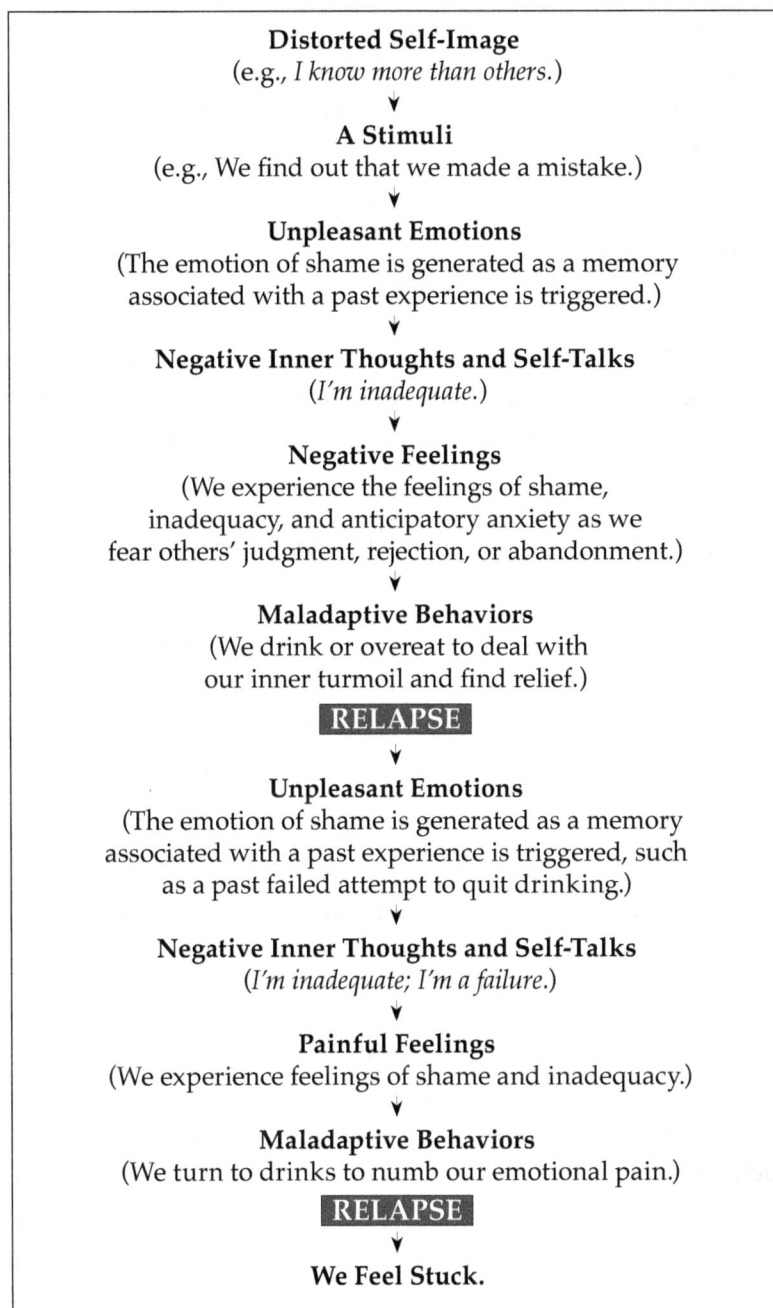

Distorted Self-Image
(e.g., *I know more than others.*)
▼
A Stimuli
(e.g., We find out that we made a mistake.)
▼
Unpleasant Emotions
(The emotion of shame is generated as a memory
associated with a past experience is triggered.)
▼
Negative Inner Thoughts and Self-Talks
(*I'm inadequate.*)
▼
Negative Feelings
(We experience the feelings of shame,
inadequacy, and anticipatory anxiety as we
fear others' judgment, rejection, or abandonment.)
▼
Maladaptive Behaviors
(We drink or overeat to deal with
our inner turmoil and find relief.)
RELAPSE
▼
Unpleasant Emotions
(The emotion of shame is generated as a memory
associated with a past experience is triggered, such
as a past failed attempt to quit drinking.)
▼
Negative Inner Thoughts and Self-Talks
(*I'm inadequate; I'm a failure.*)
▼
Painful Feelings
(We experience feelings of shame and inadequacy.)
▼
Maladaptive Behaviors
(We turn to drinks to numb our emotional pain.)
RELAPSE
▼
We Feel Stuck.

✿ ✿ ✿

On the other hand, when we mainly interact with an ideal environment (i.e., enlightened parents or such parental figures as siblings) during the early years of our childhood, then we tend to accumulate rewarding experiences and pleasant emotions (e.g., joy, love, and pride).

In such a case, we learn and develop healthy behaviors and coping strategies to express ourselves, deal with our painful emotions in times of stress, and build resilience.

In other words, as well-adjusted children raised in a perfect environment, we gain the ability to face problems, take responsibility for our wrongdoings, and resolve problems in an effective manner.

In such a situation, we transition into adulthood and face the real world as confident, resilient, and empowered adults.

As resilient individuals, when the neurons in the limbic area of our brain become triggered in times of stress (e.g., setbacks and challenging situations), our brain remembers rewarding outcomes and positive emotions (e.g., hope and aspiration).

These constructive emotions bring about positive internal thoughts and dialogues (e.g., *I can deal with the harsh truth*). In turn, our healthy mindset drives healthy responses and effective coping strategies (Figure 6).

Figure 7 on Page 52 illustrates how such a constructive pathway in our brain empowers us to regain a sense of control over our behaviors, overcome setbacks, fight temptations and short-term gratifications, and maintain our healthy lifestyle in such challenging times.

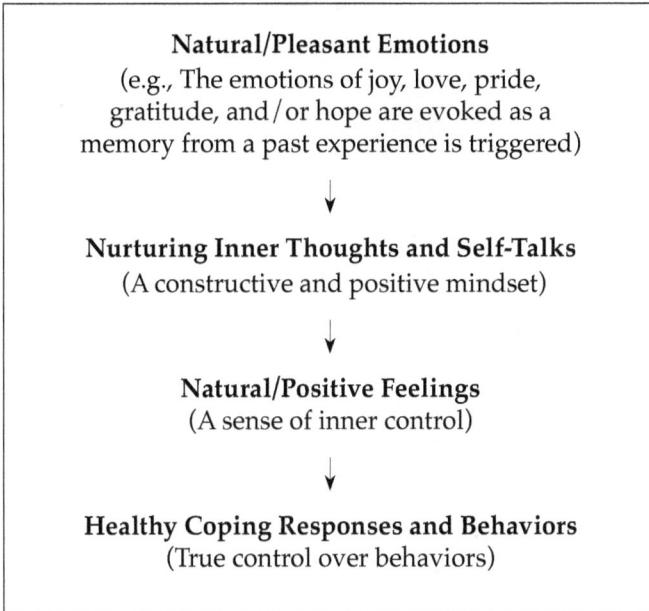

Figure 6

Natural/Pleasant Emotions
(e.g., The emotions of joy, love, pride,
gratitude, and/or hope are evoked as a
memory from a past experience is triggered)

↓

Nurturing Inner Thoughts and Self-Talks
(A constructive and positive mindset)

↓

Natural/Positive Feelings
(A sense of inner control)

↓

Healthy Coping Responses and Behaviors
(True control over behaviors)

Figure 7

Resilience

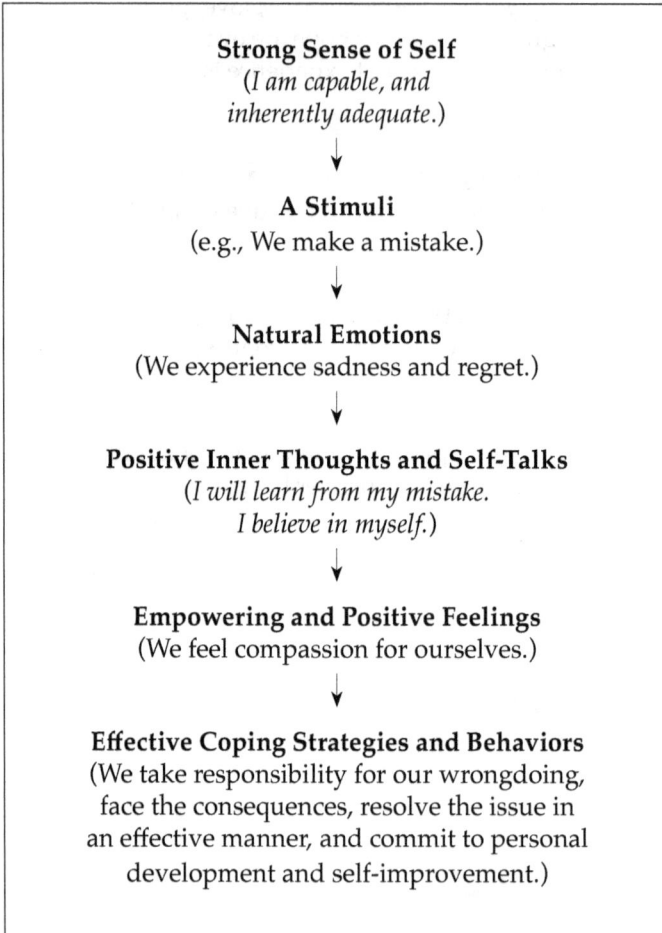

Strong Sense of Self
(*I am capable, and
inherently adequate.*)
↓

A Stimuli
(e.g., We make a mistake.)
↓

Natural Emotions
(We experience sadness and regret.)
↓

Positive Inner Thoughts and Self-Talks
(*I will learn from my mistake.
I believe in myself.*)
↓

Empowering and Positive Feelings
(We feel compassion for ourselves.)
↓

Effective Coping Strategies and Behaviors
(We take responsibility for our wrongdoing,
face the consequences, resolve the issue in
an effective manner, and commit to personal
development and self-improvement.)

In this imperfect world, as young children, the majority of us don't have the opportunity to grow up in an ideal environment.

Consequently, we may form a flawed mindset that hinders us from reaching our full potential.

However, through changing our internal thoughts and self-talks (i.e., gaining *inner control*), we can alter the way we perceive ourselves, the world around us, and the experiences we have. In turn, this altered mindset empowers us to *gain control* over our behaviors.

As discussed earlier in this book, *human development is a continual process that happens over a lifetime*: As we interact with a constructive environment (e.g., enlightened and positive people and social network) we change and better ourselves. In turn, our environment improves and changes.

Since we are no longer enslaved to the old maladaptive ways of thinking, feeling, and behaving, we will be free to make better choices, maintain a healthy lifestyle, and reach total wellness.

6

EMPOWERING INNER THOUGHTS AND SELF-TALKS

Figure 8 outlines a set of empowering internal thoughts and dialogues that is generated by *an empowering and constructive mindset* (i.e., a mindset that is gained in the process of personal growth and transformation).

🌊 🌊 🌊

Figure 8

A Learned Mindset

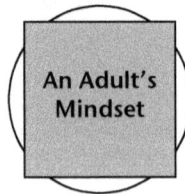

An Adult's Mindset

I'm secure; I am good enough.
I'm strong; I am not helpless, powerless, or stuck.
I'm separate; I have healthy personal boundaries.
I am free; I have choices.

I'm resilient; I can face the truth, overcome setbacks and challenges, and regain my inner control.
I'm self-disciplined; I can regulate my emotions and control my impulses and temptations.

Figure 8

A Learned Mindset (Cont'd)

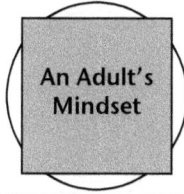

An Adult's Mindset

*I'm empathetic; I can understand and relate to
the feelings and experiences of other people.
I'm forgiving; I can let go of my anger
and reach inner calmness.
I'm giving; I have a purpose greater than myself.*

*I'm proactive; I can reach my full potential.
I'm ethical and conscientious; I am responsible towards
myself, other people, animals, and my environment.*

*I believe in myself; I am real and live an authentic life.
I'm realistic; I'm always a work-in-progress.*

*As a mature adult:
It is my responsibility to meet my basic human needs;
I am responsible for my own shelter and food.*

*I'm responsible for my own physical and
emotional health and well-being.*

*It is my responsibility to
acknowledge and affirm myself.*

*It is my responsibility to resolve my own
negative feelings and problems.*

*It is my responsibility to protect and defend my
basic human rights; I'm responsible for defining and
maintaining my personal boundaries.*

Figure 8

A Learned Mindset (Cont'd)

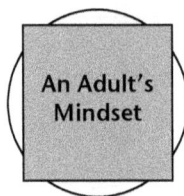

An Adult's
Mindset

I'm responsible for the choices and decisions that I make.

I'm responsible for my own happiness.

7

CONSTRUCTIVE
COMMUNICATIONS AND BEHAVIORS

This chapter lists a set of effective and constructive behaviors that are driven by empowering inner thoughts and self-talks.

*An empowering and constructive mindset that is based on
'logical principles, free will, and virtues'
drives healthy actions and positive change
and motivates us to
engage in responsible self-care,
attain total wellness, and
enjoy rewarding experiences.*

🪶 🪶 🪶

» Since we are understanding, we accept our humanness: without being enabling, we forgive ourselves for our own mistakes. As we extend our empathy towards others, we accept other people's humanness and without condoning their maladaptive behaviors, we forgive them for their wrongdoings towards us.

» We engage in *responsible* self-care while being mindful of the needs of others individuals.

» Since we have a strong sense of our *self* (self-integrity), we stay true to our own positive values and healthy beliefs.

» Being self-confident, we don't have a need to be right or win arguments in order to feel worthy; As a result, we don't dismiss other people's realities, engage in power struggles, or become argumentative.

🪶 🪶 🪶

» We communicate in an assertive manner:

- We express our *true* feelings, thoughts, needs, desires, and expectations:
  - ✓ Directly (person to person);
  - ✓ Spontaneously (not impulsively or reactively);
  - ✓ Naturally (without premeditation);
  - ✓ Mindfully and respectfully;
  - ✓ Clearly, openly, and sincerely; and,
  - ✓ Firmly.

- We maintain a relaxed posture and speak in a gentle tone of voice.

- We make eye contact that projects respect, confidence, strength, and kindness.

- We assume an equal posturing in our relationships.

- We speak in a non-provocative manner.

- We use 'I' statements: *'I' have a problem with this statement.*

- We listen without interrupting.

- We are impartial, flexible, and open-minded; therefore, we:
  - ✓ Listen to others without judging them.
  - ✓ Hear the opposing views while practicing tolerance.
  - ✓ Consider people's suggestions and ideas carefully.
  - ✓ Admit when we are wrong.
  - ✓ Reconsider our beliefs when we find out a different truth.

- Although we feel secure to express ourselves freely, we regulate our emotions and urges and practice self-restraint in circumstances where our freedom of expression impacts our environment in a negative way or causes suffering in others. For example, when we are feeling frustrated, we avoid making remarks that turn people against each other.

- While we are flexible, we remain strong. In other words, we are not malleable or easily controlled or influenced by others.

- Since our sense of self-value or self-worth doesn't depend upon external outcomes, we don't make poor choices to please other people. Rather, we make well-thought-out decisions that are based on logical principles, sound values, and free-will and result in positive outcomes. For example, we choose a relationship partner based on such criteria as genuine love, mutual respect, trust, good communication, and whether we are at *our best true* self when we are with the individual, not based on what the people in our social circle think.

- We create a positive and healthy environment for ourselves by including people in our lives who inspire us to be the best we can be.

- We create a positive and healthy environment for other people through leading by example.

- We are mindful of our surrounding physical environment and take logical measures to be eco-friendly.

🌊° 🌊° 🌊°

» We resolve our conflicts effectively:
   - Since we remain strong and secure, we address issues as they arise in a rational, calm, and effective manner; therefore, we don't bottle up, hold grudges, develop a victim mentality, or form grievance stories.

   - We remain unaffected by other people's reactivity or judgments of us because we are self-confident. Thus, we don't *react*; rather, we *act*. For example, instead of reacting and isolating ourselves, we would choose to cut off from our family, significant other, or others only when we are certain that it is a well-thought-out *action*.

❦ ❦ ❦

» We are conscientious and responsible; therefore:

- ○ Instead of becoming annoyed when people think, feel, behave in certain ways, we own our negative feelings and work towards building tolerance, acceptance, and empathy.

- ○ Instead of being demanding, we make requests.

- ○ Instead of jumping to conclusions, judging people, or taking things personally, we ask questions, become enlightened, and make observations.

- ○ Instead of distorting our reality and seeing things the way we wish them to be (avoidance), we face the harsh truth.

- ○ Being realistic, we make sensible goals and then do our best to work towards progression, not perfection.

> *We make realistic goals and then work towards progression, not perfection.*

❦ ❦ ❦

The Outcomes:

» A strong sense of self:
» A positive self-image and self-identity
» Healthy and rewarding relationships
» Healthy lifestyle and responsible self-care
» Optimal physical, emotional, and mental health

PART IV

A SUPPORTIVE, REALISTIC,
AND LOGICAL MINDSET

"Would you please indulge me for a moment and consider this scenario:

Your loved one is sleepwalking. You decide to rouse them because you are concerned that they would fall down the stairs and get hurt. First, you call their name softly. They don't wake up. You call them a bit louder. No use. You gently guide them away from the staircase. To no avail. Fearing for their safety, you lightly and tenderly slap them on the face. Of course, they feel the pain but what you did helped them wake up and stay safe.

🐦 🐦 🐦

Now, let us ask ourselves: What would be a better choice: Appeasing our loved ones and sparing their feelings by distorting (i.e., sugarcoating) or disguising a harsh truth? (Of course, this way they would like us more.) Or, staying true to them by sharing the truth in a direct, straight-forward, but non-judgmental, manner? (Of course, this way we may risk hurting their feelings and making them feel resentful.)

🐦 🐦 🐦

Sometimes, to build ourselves up, we may have to first tear down the defective house that was built for us in the early years of our childhood.

However, many of us live on autopilot and may not realize that the house we've been living in is in fact defective.

Sometimes, we may need to hear this harsh truth directly, straightforwardly, and in a forthright manner so that we gain awareness, rebuild, and better ourselves.

Naturally then, to reconstruct a house that would reflect a healthier image of our 'self' may be a painful task to accomplish.

However, we can heal our painful emotions. We can take on the challenging task of transformation. We can form a healthy sense of our 'self'. We go through this difficult process because we deserve to live a fulfilled life.

'What you resist, persists.' —Carl Jung
'What you feel, you can heal.' —John Gray

What do you think? Shall we have faith in each other and be true to one another? Shall we share together the tools that have helped us build a healthier self-image without fearing each other's judgment, rejection, or abandonment?

Believe in Yourself;
Believe in Everyone.

Become Enlightened by Gaining Insight;
Enlighten Others by Expressing Yourself."

> *"It takes great courage to tell the truth.*
> *It takes even more courage to accept the truth."*
> *—Anonymous*

8

PERSPECTIVE

The following viewpoints will serve as the foundation for the nurturing inner thoughts and self-talks that are presented in Chapter 9.

🐦 🐦 🐦

When we measure our value or worth as a person based on constructive and healthy principles, then we view ourselves favorably (Figure 9). This positive self-image generates feelings of compassion and drives behaviors that promote responsible and consistent self-care.

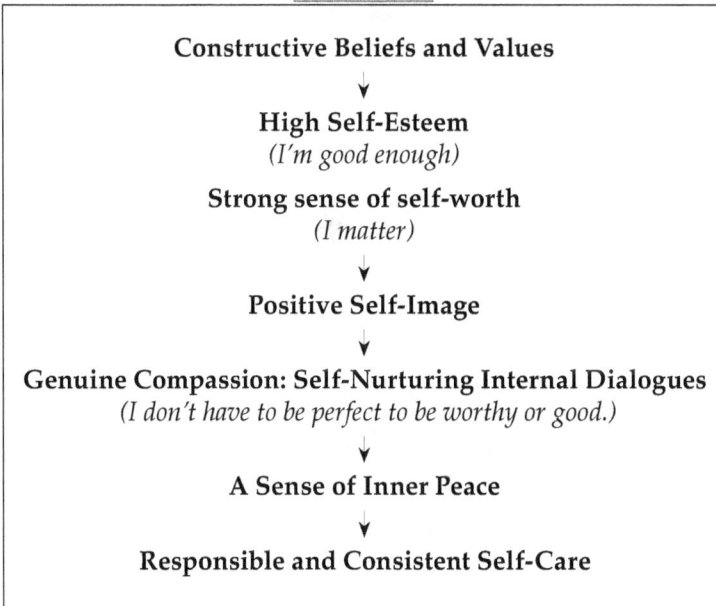

Figure 9

Constructive Beliefs and Values
↓
High Self-Esteem
(I'm good enough)

Strong sense of self-worth
(I matter)
↓
Positive Self-Image
↓
Genuine Compassion: Self-Nurturing Internal Dialogues
(I don't have to be perfect to be worthy or good.)
↓
A Sense of Inner Peace
↓
Responsible and Consistent Self-Care

On the other hand, when we measure our value or worth as a person based on flawed principles, then we may view ourselves in a distorted manner.

This distorted perception can lead to negative emotional experiences and loss of self-regard and self-compassion. In such a case, we may mindlessly engage in self-destructive behaviors to relieve our emotional suffering (Figure 10).

Figure 10

Flawed Beliefs and Values
↓
Low Self-Esteem
(I'm not good enough)

Low Self-Worth
(I don't matter)
↓
Distorted Self-Image
↓
Lack of Self-Compassion Leads to Self-Critical and Self-Depreciating Internal Dialogues
(e.g., I'm a failure)
↓
A Sense of Inner Turmoil
↓
Lack of Self-Care

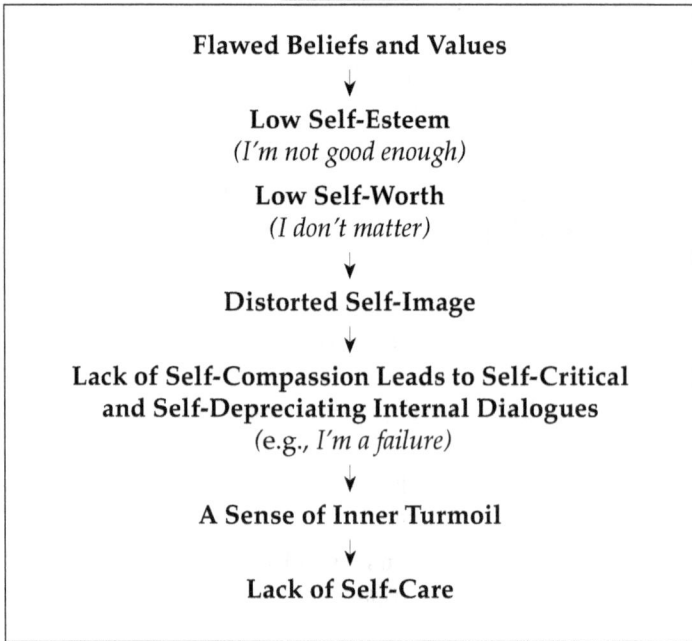

For example, as a child, we may have learned to define our value or worth based on external factors such as our appearance and physical attributes; our accomplishments; our wealth and material possessions; our social status and popularity, or other people's opinions of us.

When we remain unaware as an adult, we fail to reevaluate and change these beliefs so that we can improve ourselves and reach our full potential.

Living on autopilot, we may mindlessly harbor such negative internal dialogues as the following:

» *I'm not good or worthy if I'm not accomplished.*
» *I'm not good or worthy if I'm not wealthy.*
» *I'm not good or worthy if I'm overweight.*
» *I'm not good or worthy if I'm too tall or too short.*
» *I'm not good or worthy if I say something unwise or make a mistake.*
» *I'm not good or worthy if I don't finish my task.*
» *I'm not good or worthy if I fail my test.*
» *I'm not good or worthy if I'm divorced.*
» *I'm not good or worthy if I'm not liked by everyone.*
» *I'm not good if I say, "No!" to others.*
» *I'm not good enough because my mom says that I took after my dad.*
» *I'm narcissistic if I talk positively about myself.*
» *I'm selfish if I'm attentive to my own needs.*
» *I'm not good if I express my true opinion when it doesn't match the opinion of the majority in the group.*

When we define and evaluate ourselves based on such a faulty mindset, then we develop a distorted sense of *self* and experience many emotional problems. For example, we may become demanding, critical, and judgmental of ourselves and suffer from depression; or, we may constantly wonder or worry about what other people think of us and suffer from anxiety and mood swings.

Living our life on autopilot, we mindlessly deal and cope with our inner unrest and negative feelings either through *internalization* or *externalization*.

🌊 🌊 🌊

Internalization: When we have a poor self-image (*I am not good*), then we internalize the blame and direct the negative feelings of shame and guilt towards ourselves. As a result, we may experience the following negative outcomes:

» We become guilt-ridden.

» We suffer from self-doubt and feelings of insecurity.

» We constantly worry about how others view us.

» We neglect or dismiss our own needs as our sense of self-worth deteriorates (*I don't matter*). In order to gain a sense of inner normalcy (*I'm good*), we focus on pleasing, giving, and attending to the needs and feelings of other people, sometimes at our own expense.

» Feeling emotionally exhausted and depleted, we isolate ourselves and avoid relationships. Lacking energy and feeling depressed, we stop engaging in activities that would generally bring pleasure into our lives.

» Feeling insecure and lacking self-compassion, we become passive and allow others to cross our personal boundaries and mistreat us (e.g., we take the blame for other people's wrongdoings and therefore we enable them to project their own feelings of guilt and/or shame onto us). In such situations, we suppress our inner conflicts and bottle up our deep resentments in order to avoid others' judgment, rejection, abandonment, or their angry and retaliatory responses.

» Perceiving ourselves to be weak and defenseless, we withdraw, engage in self-pity, form a victim mentality (a state of mind in which we unconsciously wallow in self-pity as we see ourselves as a victim) and develop grievance stories (narratives that we habitually tell ourselves or others; in these stories we unconsciously refer to ourselves as the victim and others as the cause of our pain and suffering).

» When we reach our threshold, we burst with anger. However, soon after calming down, we internalize the guilt, and begin to doubt our own judgment: *It's all my fault; I'm not good . . .*

» We create a vicious cycle when we become overly apologetic, conciliatory, and passive again (Figure 11).

Figure 11

Internalization: Passivity

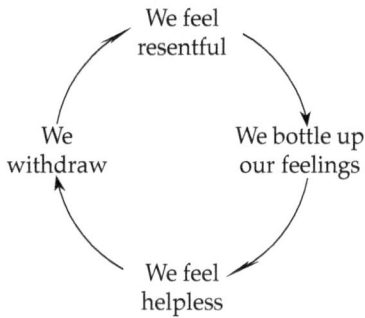

OR,

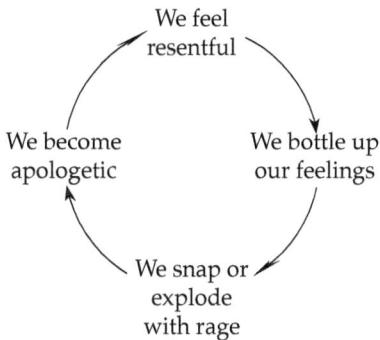

Our painful emotional experiences may further deteriorate our self-image and self-worth and lead to physical, mental, and/or emotional health problems (e.g., anxiety, depression, and autoimmune diseases).

Left unresolved, we may turn to such substances as food, alcohol, or drugs for comfort. As a result, we may struggle with dependencies, addiction, and weight issues and suffer from such chronic health problems as diabetes and cardiovascular disease.

Table 1 on the next page outlines some of our faulty patterns of thoughts and behaviors and their consequences when we internalize our negative feelings.

🐾 🐾 🐾

TABLE 1

Passivity: Internalizing Negative Feelings

Our Conscious or Subconscious Flawed Attitudes:

*I'm not worthy of being loved unless
I'm nice, helpful, and giving.*

Other people's needs are more important than mine. Poor Them!

*I 'should' be good and make others feel good in order
to be worthy of their love and approval.*

*I am powerless and helpless:
I cannot defend myself when I am faced with
people's angry or retaliatory responses. Poor Me!*

Our Passive Communications and Behaviors:

» We bottle up our negative feelings.

» We speak softly and apologetically.

» We maintain a slumped body posture.

» We make assumptions, become anxious, and withdraw when we anticipate other people's judgment, rejection, abandonment, or angry or retaliatory responses

» We have poor personal boundaries and are overly-flexible (i.e., We over-identify and over-empathize with the feelings of others; therefore, we have difficulty saying 'No' to people; feel responsible for other people's problems; fix, over function and give unsolicited advice; comply excessively to the demands of others; let other people make decisions for us; or, become overly loyal and remain committed even when the loyalty is not deserved). These behavioral tendencies enable others who have difficulty controlling their emotions to use us as a scapegoat.

» We express our feelings, opinions, needs, and wishes in an insincere manner (*insincere communications*) in order to be perceived as nice.

» We may even lack insight into ourselves (i.e., we are unaware of our own feelings, needs, and inner thoughts).

TABLE 1

Passivity: Internalizing Negative Feelings (Cont'd)

Possible Outcomes:

» Low self-worth
» Self-pity, victim mentality, and grievance stories
» Emotional dependency
» Dysfunctional relationships
» Social isolation
» Addictions/dependencies
» Suboptimal physical and/or mental health
» Financial instability
» A poor quality of life

🐦 🐦 🐦

Externalization: When we have a false sense of self-identity (i.e., I'm special; I'm better; or, I'm more capable), then our conscious or unconscious inner thoughts and self-talks may be as follows:

» *I'm not good enough if I'm not perfect. I resent people whom I perceive as being superior to me; they make me feel inferior and unimportant.*

» *I'm not good enough if I'm not right. I resent people who tell me that I'm wrong; they make me feel inferior.*

» *I'm not good enough if I make a mistake. I resent people who point out my mistake and want to help me fix it; they make me feel inferior.*

» *I'm not good enough if I don't win. I resent people who win when I lose; they make me feel inferior and unimportant.*

» *I'm not good enough if I don't have many accomplishments. I resent people who are more accomplished than I am; they make me feel inferior and unimportant.*

» *I'm not good enough if I am not admired. I resent people who criticize me; they make me feel belittled.*

» *I'm not good enough if I don't get what I want. I resent people who don't attend to my wishes; they make me feel unimportant.*

» *I'm not good enough if others don't like me. I resent people who dislike me; they make me feel bad and insecure about myself.*

» *I'm not good enough if I don't own luxury goods. I resent people who have more than I do; they make me feel inferior.*

As an imperfect human being, we naturally encounter many challenges and accumulate many disappointments when we harbor such a mindset. Over time, our sense of self-regard deteriorates (*I'm not good enough*) and we become shame-ridden.

Unable to deal with the unbearable feelings of shame and inadequacy, we project our negative feelings outwardly towards other people—our defense mechanism: *It's not me; others are not good enough.* As a result, we may experience the following negative outcomes:

» We constantly compare ourselves with other individuals; therefore, we often experience feelings of jealousy.

» We project our own feeling of shame and, consciously or unconsciously, victimize people whom we perceive as superior.

» Feeling insecure and inadequate, we strive for perfection to gain the approval of others.

» As we project our own unrealistic expectations onto other people, we become judgmental and critical when they don't think, feel, or behave in certain ways.

» To avoid feeling shame, we refuse to accept responsibility for our own mistakes, wrongdoings, or shortcomings; therefore, we become defensive; dismiss the realities of others; and shift the blame.

» When we are faced with setbacks or failures we, consciously or unconsciously, take out our frustration and anger on people whom we perceive as safe (i.e., vulnerable people or those closest to us).

» We become overly competitive, argue excessively, and engage in power struggles because we have an intense need to win or be right in order to prove that we are adequate.

» We develop low frustration tolerance and hypersensitivity to criticism as our negative experiences accumulate over time. As a result, we easily become defensive and generate a threat response. For example, we get offended and react in a punitive manner when we sense a slightest hint of condescension, disapproval, or criticism from others.

» As our confidence deteriorates, we seek relationships to regain affirmation and a sense of inner normalcy. This is when a downward spiral ensues: the individuals we are drawn to reinforce our faulty values and beliefs because they also suffer from a poor sense of self-identity.

» Our self-esteem further degrades and we become stuck.

When we engage in externalization, we generally express our negative feelings in the following ways:

» Overt aggression (e.g., we explode with rage and make a threat as our hidden inner thoughts and self-talks are: *I feel a sense of threat to my self-identity and self-importance. I'm being victimized. I need to defend myself.*) (Figure 12)

» Covert aggression (e.g., we become sarcastic as our hidden inner thoughts and self-talks are: *I feel a sense of threat to my self-identity and self-importance, but I'm too weak to defend myself. I feel trapped.*) (Figure 13 on Page 76)

After displaying externalizing behaviors, we may feel shame and guilt at the conscious or subconscious level. How we deal with our feelings of remorse may directly depend on how aware and awakened we are.

When we completely live on autopilot, we generally tend to deal with our feelings of remorse in a maladaptive way. For example, we may become a pleaser while, deep down, we are holding grudges and forming grievances stories; we may shift the blame and project our own feelings of shame and guilt (i.e., provoke the person to anger so that we would be justified in acting the way we did); or, we may withdraw and isolate ourselves.

Figure 12

Externalizing: Overt Aggression

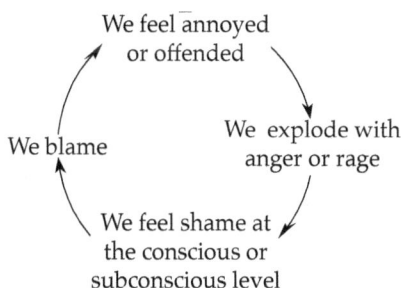

We feel annoyed or offended

We explode with anger or rage

We feel shame at the conscious or subconscious level

We blame

Figure 13

Externalizing: Covert Aggression

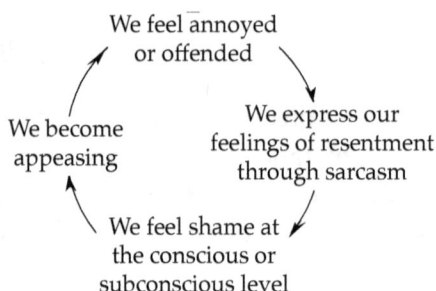

We feel annoyed
or offended

We become
appeasing

We express our
feelings of resentment
through sarcasm

We feel shame at
the conscious or
subconscious level

Our painful emotional experiences may further deteriorate our self-image and self-value and lead to fragile feelings of self-esteem, mood swings, depression, anxiety, and psychosomatic symptoms.

Left unresolved, we may turn to such substances as food, alcohol, or drugs or such adrenaline-induced activities as gambling, shopping, or video gaming for comfort. As a result, we may struggle with dependencies, addiction, weight issues, eating disorders (e.g., binge eating or anorexia), and / or financial instability and suffer from such chronic health problems as diabetes and cardiovascular disease.

Tables 2 and 3 outline some of our faulty patterns of thinking and behaving and their possible outcomes when we externalize our negative feelings.

TABLE 2

Overt Aggression: Externalizing Negative Feelings

Our Conscious or Subconscious Flawed Attitudes:

I'm deserving of receiving preferential treatment.

I have to be better than others.

I shouldn't make mistakes.

*I'm inadequate if I receive
negative feedback from people.*

*I'm not good enough if I don't get
people's approval or attention.*

*I deeply resent others who make me feel
inferior, inadequate, or unimportant.*

*I have to defend and protect myself against people who
victimize and make me feel that I'm not good enough.*

Our Aggressive Communications and Behaviors:

» We express our negative feelings in an angry, hostile, and volatile manner (e.g., we raise our voice, use "you" statements, become verbally and / or physically abusive, maintain an overbearing or intimidating posture, or make piercing eye contact)

» We control our environment through humiliation, intimidation, or domination (e.g., we make threats to get our ways or retaliate and punish those who offend us)

» We have a poor listening skill (e.g., we interrupt others frequently)

» We set and maintain rigid personal boundaries (e.g., we argue excessively or resist adopting new ideas that we haven't come up with)

» We have difficulty relating to other people's feelings and experiences (e.g., we become mindless of others' personal boundaries)

» We make poor or unethical choices (e.g., we lie or shift the blame to save face)

TABLE 2

Overt Aggression: Externalizing Negative Feelings (Cont'd)

» We take things personally, distort our reality, and respond to perceived threats to our sense of identity and self-importance (e.g., we feel belittled and therefore we become defensive when we receive a negative feedback)

Possible Outcomes:

» Low self-esteem
» Behavioral tendencies that are viewed as exploitative, demanding, or controlling by other people may lead to dysfunctional relationships and social isolation
» Low frustration tolerance that results in loss of self-control and outbursts of anger, rage, and/or violence may generate hatred and anxiety in others and result in social rejection and ostracism
» Self-pity, victim mentality, and grievance stories
» Addictions/dependencies
» Suboptimal physical and/or mental health (e.g., anxiety disorder due to fears of others' judgment, rejection, or abandonment)
» Financial instability
» A poor quality of life

TABLE 3

Covert Aggression: Externalizing Negative Feelings

Our Conscious or Subconscious Flawed Attitudes:

I have to be better than others;
I shouldn't make mistakes.

I'm inadequate if I receive negative feedback
from other people.

I'm not good enough if I don't get
people's approval or attention.

I'm good and worthy when I'm in control of my environment:
when I fix, give advice, or take care of others.

I'm deserving of receiving preferential treatment because
I give and over function for people.

I deeply resent others who victimize me and make me feel
inferior, inadequate, or unimportant.

I deeply resent people who make me feel that I don't matter;
They enrage me,

I'm too weak to stand up for myself.

I feel powerless when I face others' angry or retaliatory
responses; I feel trapped. Poor Me!

Our Passive-Aggressive Communications and Behaviors:

» We bottle up and communicate negative feelings in subtle, indirect, or non-verbal manners (e.g., we mutter, show contempt by rolling our eyes, tease, ridicule, or use sarcasm to express our feelings of resentment when we are offended)

» We control other people through using indirect or nonverbal tactics in order to deal with our own negative feelings (e.g., we yawn to control undesired conversations or badmouth those whom we resent)

» We set and maintain rigid personal boundaries through indirect resistance (e.g., we engage in defiance and power struggles to resist adopting new ideas that we haven't come up)

TABLE 3

Covert Aggression: Externalizing Negative Feelings (Cont'd)

» We use psychosomatic symptoms and/or complaints (e.g., anxiety or chest pain) to control our environment and cope with our unbearable emotions

» We take things personally, distort our reality, and respond to perceived threats to our sense of identity and self-importance (e.g., we feel belittled and therefore we become resentful and sarcastic when we receive a negative feedback)

» We compare ourselves and our loved ones with others

» We make poor or unethical choices (e.g., we lie to save face or pretend that we are cooperative while in reality we are not)

» We have difficulty relating to other people's feelings and experiences (e.g., we become mindless of others' personal boundaries, judge, criticize, give unsolicited advice, fix or tell others what they should or shouldn't do)

» We express ourselves in a confusing or insincere manner (*insincere communications*) because we fear other people's judgments, rejection, or anger (e.g., we say we are fine when we feel hurt, or we make facial expression that does not match the way we feel)

Possible Outcomes:

» Fragile self-esteem
» Self-pity, victim mentality, and grievance stories
» Behavioral tendencies, such as subtle sabotaging tactics, that are viewed as emotionally abusive may result in ostracism and dysfunctional relationships
» Explosive outbursts of anger/rage may generate hatred and anxiety in others and lead to social isolation
» Addictions/dependencies
» Suboptimal physical and/or mental health (e.g., anxiety disorder due to fears of others' judgment, rejection, or abandonment)
» Financial instability
» A poor quality of life

9

NURTURING INNER THOUGHTS
AND SELF-TALKS

This chapter presents nurturing inner thoughts and dialogues that are driven by *a supportive, realistic, and logical mindset* (i.e., a mindset that is gained through the process of personal growth and transformation).

🌀 🌀 🌀

I realize that when I define my value or worth as a person based on a set of flawed values that I learned in the early years, I swing back and forth between the states of self-congratulation (*I'm better or I'm more capable*) and self-depreciation (*I'm inferior or I'm inadequate*).

For example, when I evaluate my self-value based on how others view me, then I may develop a distorted self-image that is projected onto me by others. In this case, my self-regard and self-compassion could fluctuate from moment to moment: one day I receive attention and praise from people at work, so I like myself and feel self-confident; I may even think that I'm special or better than others. The next day, I receive negative feedback from my boss or coworkers, so I end up disliking myself and feeling inadequate and inferior.

This inner conflict confuses me, keeps me from seeing a true image of myself, and damages my sense of self-esteem. Ultimately, the lack of self-regard and self-compassion hinders me from engaging in self-care.

By contrast, when I define my value or worth as a person

based on a set of constructive and logical principles and virtues, then I become empowered to see a true image of myself: *I am an imperfect human being; I am unique and worthy of being loved; I matter. I am neither superior nor inferior to anyone.*

This more realistic and positive mindset empowers me to become more mindful, nurturing, and respectful of my own feelings, realities, and needs—an act of genuine compassion towards myself. Having a positive self-image and genuine self-compassion results in the following positive experiences and favorable outcomes in my life:

» I will experience a high level of self-confidence.

» When I feel self-assured, I will become free to pay more attention to my environment (i.e., my family, friends, co-workers, and other people).

» When I am more aware and mindful of others, I will gain more insight into them and become more understanding and tolerant.

» Having genuine empathy towards others will lead to more rewarding relationships and favorable outcomes in my life.

» As I will no longer feel compelled to please people in order to gain their approval and affirmation, I will feel liberated to make well-thought-out choices that are based on logical and constructive principles, virtues, and free-will. For example, I will choose friends or a life partner based on such criteria as shared interests and virtues, and whether they bring out the best in me.

» Living a more fulfilled life will invigorate me to engage in a more consistent and effective self-care and achieve optimal health.

❧ ❧ ❧

I realize that when I define other people's value or worth based on a set of flawed values and beliefs that I learned in the early years, I swing between the states of self-righteousness (feeling annoyance or rage) and remorse (feeling shame and/or guilt). These conflicting states of *being* damage my relationships and negatively impact my total well-being.

However, when I cultivate constructive principles, healthy values, and virtues of love and humanity, then I become empowered to see a true image of other people: As imperfect human beings, other people are unique and wor*thy of being loved as well. They matter as much as I do. They are neither superior nor inferior to me.*

This more realistic and positive mindset enables me to become more mindful, nurturing, tolerant, and respectful of the feelings, realities, and needs of others. Having genuine compassion towards people leads to such positive experiences and favorable outcomes as the following:

» Having a more positive attitude towards others will keep me from taking things personally in situations where I perceive myself as being judged or treated unfairly by them. Consequently, I will become empowered to stay non-reactive and resolve my issues more effectively.

» As I experience more rewarding relationships with my significant other, coworkers, friends, and other people in my environment, I will not face negative outcomes such as anxiety (i.e., fears of other people's judgment or rejection) that may lead to maladaptive coping behaviors.

> *Living a more fulfilled life invigorates us to engage in a more consistent and effective self-care.*

PART V

A MINDFUL, CONSCIENTIOUS,
AND EMPATHETIC MINDSET

Once an insightful person asked:
"My glass is empty. How do I nurture myself?"

She received this reply:
"Find the seeds of empathy through gaining insight into
yourself. Then, plant it, nurture it, and extend it to others.
Before long, it will nurture you back."

She took the advice and followed it through.
After a period of intense work, she shared:
"Now, my glass is full!"

10

PERSPECTIVE

The following viewpoints will serve as the foundation for the perceptive inner thoughts and self-talks that are presented in Chapter 12.

❦ ❦ ❦

When we learn to evaluate ourselves based on how other people view us, we may not only see our own image through the lens of others but also make decisions from a place of weakness, fear, and need—we feel insecure and inadequate; fear others' judgment, rejection, and abandonment; and, need other people's affirmation or attention to feel good about ourselves.

For example, in order to please and win the approval of our friends, we may make careless choices that appear as though we are being self-serving, immoral, or inconsiderate towards some others whom we perceive as safe (e.g., our loved ones). In situations like this, our mindless behaviors may convey unintended hurtful messages such as, *"You don't matter to me . . . others are more important."*

Our poor choices naturally result in negative consequences. For instance, people, who have remained unawakened and carry unhealed emotional wounds from the past, may take our behavior personally. Instead of expressing themselves and setting their limits in an effective manner of communication, they may act upon their feelings of resentment and judge, criticize, and punish us. When we remain unaware, we may be unable to relate to their experiences and understand why our behavior made them feel and react the way they did. A vicious cycle is created when we, instead of bearing responsibility for our own part in the conflict, also become reactive and externalize our negative feelings by shifting the blame onto them (Figure 14).

❧ ❧ ❧

Moreover, when we learn to evaluate ourselves based on how others perceive us, then we may develop an intense urge to be perfect (i.e., look perfect or reach perfection in everything that we do) in order to gain people's approval. In this case, we may set unrealistic and unattainable goals, avoid mistakes or failure at all cost, become rigid and harbor an all-or-none attitude, and judge ourselves severely since any deviation and inconsistency becomes intolerable to us.

Our perfectionistic mindset may lead to such maladaptive behaviors and negative consequences as the following:

» We become self-judgmental, self-critical, and self-loathing when we make a mistake.

» We become moody since we are unable to please or gain the approval of *everyone*.

» We develop depression and suffer from the feelings of despair, inadequacy, and helplessness because, as human beings, we are imperfect and inevitably face failures and setbacks.

» We develop anxiety disorders, suffer from obsessive and ruminative thinking, engage in compulsive behaviors, and become controlling because we have chronic fears of:

  ◦ Making mistakes;

  ◦ Experiencing failures; and,

  ◦ Being judged, disapproved, and rejected by others.

Figure 14

A Hypothetical Case Study

We evaluate our sense of self-value based
on how others view us.
↓
We become a people-pleaser and neglect the needs of our
spouse (referred to as X) whom we perceive as safe.
↓
X takes things personally, feels hurt
(*I'm not important; I don't matter*), and complains that
we always take him/her for granted.
↓
At the subconscious level, we also take things personally.
Feeling judged and criticized (*I'm not a good spouse . . . I'm
inadequate*), we shift the blame and project our
own feelings of shame and guilt onto X:
"You are being needy and demanding."
↓
X internalizes the shame and guilt that is projected onto
him/her and experiences the conflicting feelings of
guilt/self-doubt (*I was bad*) and resentment.
↓
X becomes conciliatory and appeasing while
he/she represses the feelings of resentment
at the conscious or subconscious level.
↓
X becomes emotionally distant.
↓
Remaining unaware, we feel rejected:
I'm not good enough.
↓
Over time, our self-image and sense of
self-esteem deteriorates.

Being on autopilot, we unconsciously create the vicious cycle of self-entrapment when we resort to our primitive defense mechanisms to deal with our painful emotions. For example, in a situation in which we are faced with the consequences of our mistakes, the resultant feelings of shame and inadequacy trigger a set of automatic responses that were conditioned in us during childhood, such as avoidance (i.e., we distract ourselves by pursuing pleasure) or projection (i.e., we shift the blame). These automatic behaviors, which protected and insulated us from experiencing further emotional pain as children, become maladaptive later in life since their negative consequences reinforce our poor self-image (Figure 15).

❦ ❦ ❦

Furthermore, when we struggle with perfectionism, we may unconsciously project our own values onto others. For example, we may assume that people are evaluating and judging us based on the same extremely high expectations. When time after time we naturally fail to please everyone and live up to our own unrealistic and high expectations, we come to stop believing in ourselves. This lack of self-confidence intensifies our emotional pain in the following ways:

» We become shame-ridden because we feel like a failure. Thus, we lose motivation and slip into a state of apathy.

» Since we lack trust in our own judgments, we become indecisive and have difficulty making hard decisions.

» Lacking faith in ourselves and our own abilities makes us unwilling to work hard, do our best, and challenge ourselves. For example, we may procrastinate or unconsciously look for distractions to postpone or avoid challenging tasks that cause stress and anxiety.

Figure 15

A Hypothetical Case Study

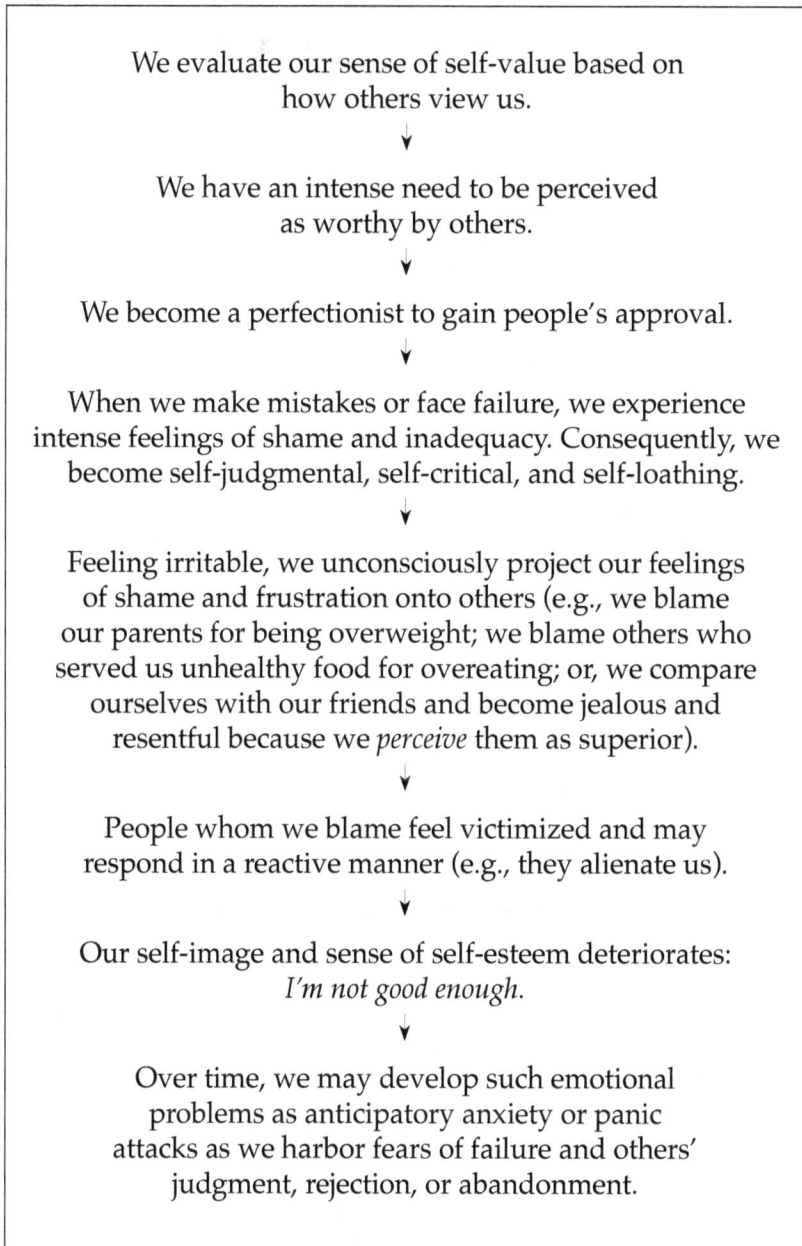

We evaluate our sense of self-value based on
how others view us.

↓

We have an intense need to be perceived
as worthy by others.

↓

We become a perfectionist to gain people's approval.

↓

When we make mistakes or face failure, we experience
intense feelings of shame and inadequacy. Consequently, we
become self-judgmental, self-critical, and self-loathing.

↓

Feeling irritable, we unconsciously project our feelings
of shame and frustration onto others (e.g., we blame
our parents for being overweight; we blame others who
served us unhealthy food for overeating; or, we compare
ourselves with our friends and become jealous and
resentful because we *perceive* them as superior).

↓

People whom we blame feel victimized and may
respond in a reactive manner (e.g., they alienate us).

↓

Our self-image and sense of self-esteem deteriorates:
I'm not good enough.

↓

Over time, we may develop such emotional
problems as anticipatory anxiety or panic
attacks as we harbor fears of failure and others'
judgment, rejection, or abandonment.

» Since we struggle with self-discipline, we either quit soon after starting a demanding task or withdraw all together.

» As negative experiences accumulate over time, we become pessimistic and experience the feelings of hopelessness, helplessness, and sadness. Thus, we end up suffering from depression.

» At the subconscious level, we may avoid difficult situations through transforming our painful emotions into physical symptoms. Thus, we suffer from psychosomatic disorders.

» We become self-focused and end up under-functioning (e.g., we break our commitments). Consequently, we may have poor interpersonal relationships.

» We may withdraw to avoid painful emotional experiences. For example, we stop engaging in social activities in order to avoid people's judgments that generate the unconscious inner thought, *I'm not good enough.* Consequently, we experience social isolation.

❦ ❦ ❦

When we adopt a perfectionistic mindset to gain others' affirmation or approval, then we may impose our high expectations on people in our immediate environment (e.g., our coworkers or those individuals whom we falsely perceive as our extension, such as our partner, spouse, children, or parents). (See Figure 16.)

In this case, we may become self-righteous (i.e., demand that others think, feel, and behave in certain ways), unforgiving (i.e., hold grudges), and punitive (i.e., become inappropriately harsh when others make mistakes). For instance, when we evaluate our children based on perfection and hold them accountable to our unrealistic expectations—in particular, in the areas of appearance, performance, or accomplishment, then:

Figure 16

A Hypothetical Case Study

We have developed a perfectionistic mindset.

↓

We unconsciously impose our values on those closest to us, such as a loved one (referred to as X), whom we falsely perceive as our extension.

↓

Although we may be loving, we become controlling: we insist that X thinks, feels, or behaves in certain ways that are acceptable to the norms of the environment we live in (i.e., our society or social group).

↓

We become annoyed, judgmental, and critical when X doesn't meet our unrealistic expectations. For example, we may criticize or make negative remarks about X's weight or appearance.

↓

X takes things personally (*I am not good enough the way I am*), becomes resentful, and externalizes his/her feelings of shame and inadequacy in a passive-aggressive manner (e.g., X engages in power-struggles).

↓

We take things personally, feel victimized, and become reactive (e.g., we give the cold shoulder and/or badmouth X).

↓

X feels victimized and responds in a retaliatory manner (e.g., X becomes defiant and rebellious).

↓

Over time, our sense of self-esteem deteriorates (*I'm inadequate*) while X develops a poor sense of self and suffers from such problems as anxiety and eating disorders (e.g., binge eating).

» We may become inflexible and rigid (i.e., become intolerant of flaws, deviations, and imperfections).

» We may become judgmental, critical, and demanding (i.e., insist that they *should* follow our views because we know better and they don't).

» We may experience anxiety and feel helpless and therefore we become controlling (i.e., shame or guilt them into conformity).

Although we have good intentions and a loving attitude towards our children (we may even have a *general permissive* parenting style), this flawed mindset, which we have developed in the early years of our childhood, can lead to harmful psychological problems in our children (e.g., loss of confidence, indecisiveness, anxiety, obsessive-compulsive tendencies, and, eating disorders).

🐾 🐾 🐾

When we learn to evaluate ourselves based on how others perceive us, then we may become preoccupied by such factors as how much attention, approval, or praise we receive from people (Figure 17). In this case, our experiences may be as follows:

» We become needy and engage in attention-seeking behaviors that defeat our purpose and drive people away.

» We constantly compare ourselves with others and become competitive and jealous.

» We give up our autonomy and develop an emotional dependency: Since our self-esteem, self-confidence, and happiness depends on an external source (i.e., other people's attention, approval, or affirmation), we have a constant urge to surround ourselves with people or be involved in relationships that affirm us and help us reach a sense of inner normalcy (i.e., *I'm worthy . . . I'm important . . . I'm good enough . . .*). Moreover, we may give up our individuality and separateness and become a people pleaser to gain other people's approval. Therefore, instead of making choices that are based on *free-will and logical, reasonable, and ethical principles,* we may make

Figure 17

A Hypothetical Case Study

We evaluate our sense of self-value based on how much
attention, approval, or praise we receive from others.

↓

We become preoccupied with fitting in
and being liked at work.

↓

We engage in attention-seeking behaviors and become
mindless or callous towards some coworkers whom
we perceive as unpopular or inferior.

↓

Other coworkers, who think we are selfish, avoid us.

↓

Since we lack insight into ourselves and others, we
take things personally and think: *I'm not good enough.*

↓

Feeling insecure, we compare ourselves and develop
feelings of jealousy and animosity towards a coworker
(referred to as X) who is more popular.
We externalize our feelings of inadequacy and
resentment by treating X with hostility.

↓

Other coworkers judge and criticize us as being mean;
they reject us and give us the cold shoulder.

↓

Holding grudges, we denigrate and badmouth X to elevate
or justify ourselves: *I'm good; X is the bad one.*

↓

Our negative and hostile attitude
further drives others away.

↓

Our self-image and sense of self-esteem
deteriorates: *I am a loser.*

decisions that are based on the opinions of people in our social group. In such cases, we are likely to make poor choices and face negative consequences. Over time, we stop believing in our own judgment and decision-making abilities and become dependent on others to make decisions for us.

» We become self-serving, pretentious, and exclusionary: in order to gain others' admiration or approval, we may become preoccupied with such external factors as our physical appearance, accomplishments, or social and financial status. To elevate ourselves and get the admiration of others, we may form *many* friendships and *work hard* to please our friends. Additionally, we may seek out friendship with those whom we perceive as popular/superior while excluding those whom we have disdain for because we consider them to be unpopular/inferior.

» We become moody and experience such conflicting feelings as love/hate. This is because our mood and feelings swing as our experience with people changes. For example, we are in a good mood and feel loving towards others when we receive their attention, praise, or approval; we become depressed and feel contempt or hatred when we receive disapproval or negative feedback from them.

» We suffer from social anxiety as we constantly fear people's disapproval, judgment, rejection, or abandonment.

» We lead an unfulfilled life and develop depression because:
  ◦ We cannot possibly please everyone; therefore, we feel hopeless and sad.
  ◦ We over-function for people to please them; thus, we often end up feeling taken advantage of, used, and trapped. Since we neglect and under-function for our-selves, we feel emotionally depleted.
  ◦ We are emotionally dependent on others; therefore, we often feel helpless and unfulfilled.

» We easily become offended when we receive negative feedback from others.

» We become demanding and resentful and alienate people when we don't receive the approval or attention that we expect.

» In order to elevate ourselves, we denigrate, ridicule, tease, or badmouth people and further put a strain on our relationships.

» Lacking insight into ourselves, we fail to see our own part in our emotional suffering; therefore, we constantly feel stuck.

» Feeling helpless, powerless, and trapped, we wallow in self-pity and develop a victim mentality (perceive ourselves as a victim).

» Over time, we form grievance stories that we tell ourselves and others . In these stories, we shift the blame and perceive ourselves as the victim who needs to be helped, defended, and pitied. Subconsciously, we may use our grievance stories to evoke sympathy and get the attention that we need to feel a sense of inner normalcy.

❦ ❦ ❦

Similarly, when we measure our self-value based on such external factors as our appearance, financial status, or social class, then we develop a flawed mindset that generates emotional pain and drives maladaptive behaviors (our defense mechanisms).

For example, we may constantly compare ourselves with others; become self-focused, competitive and jealous; and, externalize our feelings of inadequacy and shame by victimizing people whom we perceive as superior or scapegoating those whom we consider *safe* (e.g., people closest to us) or *easy* (e.g., unpopular people whom we perceive as inferior).

As other unawakened people take our behaviors personally, we may face their judgment, rejection, abandonment, or angry and retaliatory reactions.

Living on autopilot, we create a downward spiral when we resort to such defense mechanisms as avoidance to deal with our emotional suffering.

❦ ❦ ❦

On the other hand, when we learn to measure our *self-worth* based on how much we *matter* to other people, then we may constantly focus on giving, helping, and serving the needs of others—even when those individuals are able to help themselves (Figure 18).

In seeking others' validation that *we are good and worthy of being loved*, we may become excessively attentive to people, specifically, to those who are closest to us.

As we *over-identify* and *over-empathize* with the feelings and experiences of others, rather than with those of our own, we may overlook, neglect, and even sacrifice our needs for theirs.

In such situations, we may enable people to under-function for themselves and become emotionally and/or physically dependent on us. (This may gratify our deep-seated desire of *being needed*: *I'm important to them; therefore, I matter!*)

Moreover, our over-functioning may embolden others to inadvertently become self-focused and inattentive and careless towards us. The disparity between giving and taking creates imbalanced and one-sided relationships and leads to undesired outcomes for everyone involved.

The following outlines some of the challenges that we may face (and create for others) when we remain unaware and continue to lead such one-sided relationships:

Figure 18

A Hypothetical Case Study

We evaluate our worth as a person based on how
much we matter to other people.

↓

After having a heated argument with a coworker
at work, our spouse (referred to as X) comes
home feeling frustrated.

↓

X starts venting his/her anger.

↓

We *over*-identify with X's thoughts
and *over*-empathize with his/her feelings

↓

Needing to be helpful, we over-function:

» We analyze X's actions: how X *should have* resolved the
issue with the coworker;

» We give advice and *insist* that X *should* follow it; and,

» Attempting to alleviate X's emotional distress, we
minimize the significance of the event and mindlessly
dismiss X's feelings by saying, *"You're overthinking it . . .*
You're getting all upset over nothing . . . "

↓

X, who suffers from a low sense of self-value and tends to
seek our affirmation to feel adequate, takes things personally:
I'm being judged; my realities and feelings are being dismissed . . .
My spouse doesn't believe in me or my abilities to resolve my
own problems. He/she thinks that I'm inadequate . . .

↓

Feeling resentful and belittled (*I'm not good enough*),
X becomes reactive and externalizes his/her feelings
in an aggressive manner: *"You are so insensitive . . .*
You have no empathy . . . You always judge me . . .
You think you know it all."

↓

(Cont'd on Page 102)

Figure 18

A Hypothetical Case Study (Cont'd)

↓

Lacking insight into ourselves or X, we take
things personally and feel hurt and unappreciated:
*I am never appreciated; I can't help . . . I'm useless . . .
I'm inadequate as a spouse . . .*

↓

We develop anxiety (i.e., we fear X's
rejection or abandonment) and bottle up
our feelings of resentment.

↓

We become distant and form a triangle to relieve our
feelings of anxiety, helplessness, and resentment
(e.g., we use our children as our
confidant and badmouth X).

↓

After calming down, we develop feelings of
guilt and self-doubt and become
apologetic and conciliatory.

↓

Needing X's validation that we matter,
we continue to over-function even when X is
able to help himself/herself.

↓

Since we seldom receive the acknowledgment that
we need in order to feel a sense of inner normalcy,
our sense of self-worth deteriorates over time:
I'm not worthy of being loved; I don't matter.

As time goes on, X's sense of self-
value deteriorates:
*I can't make my spouse happy . . .
I'm not good enough . . .*

» Lacking insight into ourselves and others, we take things personally and feel unloved, unappreciated, used, taken for granted, unfulfilled, and resentful.

» As time goes on, we become physically and/or emotionally exhausted and feel drained.

» Being on autopilot, we become reproachful and demand that others treat us the way we treat them. While genuinely believing that we have good intentions, we cross people's personal boundaries in order to *fix/change* them and improve our relationships.

» Our maladaptive coping behavior triggers those who have also remained unawakened: They take things personally; feel judged, belittled, controlled, and resentful; and, respond in a reactive manner (e.g., they externalize their negative feelings by displaying overt or covert aggression).

» We feel hurt, angry, and/or enraged when we face other people's reactivity, instead of receiving their appreciation or acknowledgment, which we had unrealistically anticipated to receive.

» Consequently, we react and externalize our negative feelings. For example, we may express ourselves in an aggressive manner (e.g., we snap, burst into anger, and become critical and punitive); or, we may become passive-aggressive and control in a covert manner (e.g., we give the silent treatment or badmouth them behind their back).

» This dynamic becomes even more dysfunctional when we calm down and experience the feelings of self-doubt, guilt, and anxiety (i.e., due to fear of others' judgment, rejection, or abandonment).

» Since we rely on external validation to think that *we are good and worthy of being loved*, we become conciliatory and apologetic.

» We create a downward vicious cycle when we revert to our old pattern (i.e., we continue to over-function in our relationships and face the same interpersonal issues):

○ Feeling helpless, powerless, and trapped, we wallow in self-pity and develop a victim mentality (perceive ourselves as a victim).

○ We form grievance stories that we tell ourselves and other people. In these stories, we shift the blame and perceive ourselves as the victim who needs to be helped, defended, and pitied. Subconsciously, we may use our grievance stories to evoke sympathy, get the acknowledgement that we are good and worthy of being loved, and reach an inner normalcy.

○ Lacking insight into ourselves, we fail to see our own part in our emotional suffering. Feeling stuck, we may resort to such defense mechanisms as avoidance to deal with our emotional suffering.

For further reading on these subjects and finding strategies to overcome the feelings of resentment refer to *Accountability and Empowerment*.

11

EMOTIONAL HEALING:
EMPATHY AND FORGIVENESS

Having faced *our truth* and become aware of our deeply-ingrained flawed beliefs that have generated our faulty character traits, we may now be experiencing some degree of inner turmoil: Perhaps, some repressed memories from the past have resurfaced; Maybe certain painful emotions, such as shame, guilt, anger, or resentment, have generated.

This chapter explores a state of true *emotional healing.*

🐚 🐚 🐚

Emotional healing is a *process* that happens over time. It brings about a sense of liberation, general well-being, empowerment, and inner peace.

This process begins with gaining insight into ourselves and developing self-empathy: when we discover *our truth* and make sense of it all (i.e., why we do what we do that leads to painful emotions and negative outcomes), then we come to understand our experiences and see *the truth: our humanness.* This is when we become empowered to forgive ourselves for our own mistakes and wrongdoings.

Accepting our human imperfections helps us connect to other people, relate to their experiences, and understand their feelings. This is when we become empowered to forgive others and reach true and lasting emotional healing.

Let us delve deeper into this premise by first exploring the concepts of *empathy* and *forgiveness.*

🐚 🐚 🐚

Empathy is a state of mind that empowers us to *relate* to one's experience and *understand* the feelings that this experience generates in that individual. This state of mind is produced through the process of non-judgmental observations and reflection.

For example, we cultivate and develop an empathetic mindset towards others when we put ourselves in their place and see things through their eyes.

Although we may not agree with their reality (i.e., their perception of events), our non-judgmental observations generate valuable knowledge about their patterns of thoughts, feelings, and behaviors and help us understand *their truth*: how they perceive events, why they see them in certain ways, and what type of feelings their perception generates in them that trigger them to behave the way they do.

As we make sense of it all and understand why others think, feel, and behave the way they do, we can connect with them at the human level: we can relate to their experiences, understand their feelings, accept their humanness, and develop compassion for them as a person (Figure 19).

We show this *understanding* and *acceptance* (empathy) by acknowledging people's feelings in a respectful and supportive manner—even when we could not condone their attitudes or behaviors.

Similarly, we cultivate and develop an empathetic mindset towards ourselves when we connect with our *self* in a non-judgmental manner. Our mindfulness and self-observation helps us discover our *inner thoughts that generate our feelings and drive our behaviors.*

When we make sense of our experience and gain an insight into ourselves, we discover *our truth*—why we think, feel, and behave the way we do.

This self-discovery helps us see and accept our humanness and become more understanding towards ourselves.

As we understand ourselves better, we become empowered to have compassion for ourselves. In such a state of mind, we can acknowledge *all* of our feelings (good or bad) in a nurturing and supportive manner—even when we could not condone our own attitudes or behaviors.

Figure 19

We put ourselves in people's place and
see things through their eyes.

↓

We make non-judgmental observations and gain
insight into how their pattern of thoughts generates
their feelings and drives their behaviors.

↓

We connect to them at the human level:
We understand their feelings.

🌼 🌼 🌼

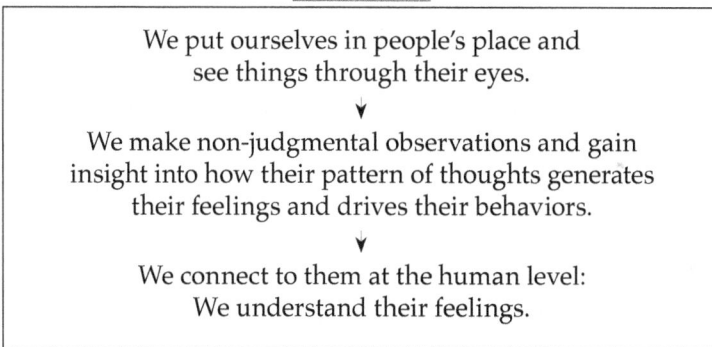

It is imperative that we make a distinction between empathy and sympathy: As discussed earlier, when we empathize with other people's feelings, we *understand* why they are thinking, feeling, and acting in a certain way, even when we cannot condone their behaviors. In this case, we are seeing and validating the individual's *total self: I hear your reality and understand your feelings. Understanding your truth enables me to see You and connect with you as a person.*

When others feel acknowledged and affirmed, they don't see themselves helpless or stuck (as we may all normally do during vulnerable times). Believing in themselves, they become empowered to see choices and improve the quality of their lives.

This is also true in regard to ourselves: when we empathize with ourselves during setbacks or mishaps, we *understand* why we are thinking, feeling, and acting in a certain way, even when we cannot condone our behaviors.

Since we acknowledge and affirm our *total self*, we don't perceive ourselves as helpless, trapped, or less than others. Now liberated from *reducing self-dialogues*, we become empowered to see choices and live a proactive life.

🖎 🖎 🖎

On the other hand, when we offer sympathy to others (when it is not warranted), we may be focusing on their misfortune—and, not so much on the person. In this case, we are not seeing or validating their *total self*; we are validating their unfortunate condition, adversity, misery, or calamity. Perhaps then, they hear: *They acknowledge the situation I am in. They pity me and feel sad that I have to face this misfortune. Perhaps, they don't believe that I can overcome this challenging situation. Perhaps, I'm pitiful and helpless. Maybe, I am inadequate and not strong enough.*

As they experience self-doubt and feel inadequate, they may come to perceive themselves as weak, helpless, and stuck. Therefore, instead of seeing choices, they may lead a passive life because they focus more on their sorrows and wallow in self-pity.

The same is true with regard to our own personal growth: during setbacks and difficult times, when we feel sorry for ourselves and engage in self-pity, then we focus on our misfortune: *Poor me!* Feeling consumed and emotionally drained, we lose the ability to see our *total self* (i.e., our inner strength). Perceiving ourselves as weak, powerless, and trapped, we deprive ourselves of the opportunity to see our options and reach our full potential.

In sum, while showing empathy fosters personal growth, offering sympathy, where it is not warranted, may inadvertently stop or limit our personal development.

🖎 🖎 🖎

Forgiveness: Perhaps, the most important step in our journey of emotional healing is forgiveness: forgiving our own past wrongdoings and then extending this forgiveness to those who have wronged us.

When we reach a state of true and genuine forgiveness, we are able to replace our emotional anguish, anger, and deep resentment with a sense of serenity, clarity, and goodwill. This is when we can learn from our past mistakes, reach inner peace, and make steady progress towards personal growth and total wellness.

Forgiveness happens through time and follows naturally after gaining insight and developing an understanding and accepting mindset towards ourselves and others (Figure 20).

While meditation, anger-management training, counseling, or religion/spirituality brings about a sense of calmness, in the absence of empathy, true forgiveness and lasting emotional healing may not be reached.

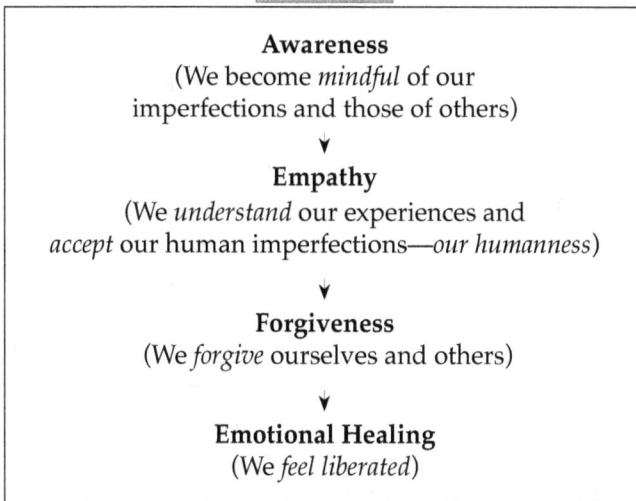

Figure 20

Awareness
(We become *mindful* of our
imperfections and those of others)
▼
Empathy
(We *understand* our experiences and
accept our human imperfections—*our humanness*)
▼
Forgiveness
(We *forgive* ourselves and others)
▼
Emotional Healing
(We *feel liberated*)

When we genuinely forgive (ourselves and others), then we may have the following experiences:

» We feel a sense of inner peace since we no longer hold grudges or experience deep-seated feelings of resentment.

» We feel more energetic as we are not spending our time ruminating over our grievances.

» We are more responsible towards ourselves and others while being more understanding (i.e., we *appropriately* hold ourselves and others accountable for mistakes and shortcomings).

» We feel a sense of liberation since we no longer see ourselves as helpless and trapped victims.

» Not being enslaved by self-pity and grievances, we are free to see our choices: We realize that, although we have no control over other people, we *have* inner control—control over our own thoughts, feelings, and behaviors.

» Since we can see all of the options that are available to us, we become empowered to lead a proactive life:

  ◦ Stay secure and strong;
  ◦ Take responsibility for our shortcomings;
  ◦ Express and defend ourselves in an appropriate and effective manner;
  ◦ Resolve issues effectively; and,
  ◦ Learn from our mistakes and commit to new ways of thinking, feeling, and behaving (e.g., we set clear, solid, and consistent boundaries in our relationships).

» We experience an improvement in our physical and mental health as forgiveness reduces cortisol level—a stress hormone that may cause the following problems:

  ◦ Psychosomatic symptoms such as dizziness, muscle aches, and backaches

- ○ Chronic physical health problems such as cardiovascular disease (e.g., high blood pressure), auto-immune disorders, and digestive problems
- ○ Mental health issues such as anxiety and depression

» We experience a more rewarding and fulfilling life as we have stable and positive relationships with our family, partner, children, friends, co-workers, and others.

※ ※ ※

On the other hand, we may not have reached a state of true and lasting forgiveness when we lead ourselves to believe that we have forgiven others while, unconsciously, we use such defense mechanisms of avoidance or suppression to deal with our feelings of resentments. In such a case:

» We enable ourselves to make the same mistakes because we avoid facing *the truth.*

» We enable others to abuse or violate our rights as we suppress, deny, or distort the reality that we were wronged in order to rationalize or justify our passivity.

» We may comfort ourselves with such substances as food or alcohol or with such behaviors as compulsive shopping or cleaning; or, we may take medications to help us deal with our depressed moods and feelings of anxiety. Thus, we may falsely believe that we are emotionally healed or that we are in healthy relationships while, in reality, we are not.

» We lead a passive and unfulfilled life: Instead of expressing our feelings in an assertive manner, we repress our emotions and may even internalize the blame, experience the feelings of shame, guilt, and self-doubt, and become self-critical.

» We create a downward spiral, when we over-empathize and for people who choose to remain unawakened (i.e., fail to offer an apology or commit to new ways of being). In doing so, we under-function for ourselves (i.e., we fail to empathize and identify with our own realities and feelings) and over function for others (i.e., we enable others to treat us poorly).

In such situations, we naturally get hurt over and over again. Over time, we end up feeling powerless, stuck, and emotionally dependent on people whom we have enabled to externalize their negative feelings and treat us poorly—people whom we enabled to remain unawakened.

🐾 🐾 🐾

As discussed previously, through gaining awareness and developing empathy, we come to accept our humanness. However, an accepting, understanding, and nurturing mindset does not result in living a passive life and facing repeated setbacks or getting hurt time after time. In other words, when we are passive and don't hold ourselves or others accountable for wrongdoings, then our enabling behavior could only result in negative consequences.

When we lead a proactive life, we don't stick by those who have wronged us and don't bear responsibility for their wrongdoings. Nevertheless, we will choose to forgive them. We do so because we deserve to experience the inner peace and the sense of liberation that forgiveness offers us.

Moreover, we choose to forgive because our own logical and empathetic mindset and compassionate heart empower us to connect and relate to people and accept their humanness.

In sum, even in situations in which it feels impossible to forgive a troubled person who has victimized and wronged us, we try our best to forgive because we may see the truth in what Buddha said: *"Holding on to anger is like grasping a hot coal with the intent of throwing it at someone else; you are the one who gets burned."*

🐾 🐾 🐾

To summarize, we reach emotional healing as we go through the following steps:

» We make non-judgmental self-observation;

» We identify our true emotions and inner thoughts;

» Our self-awareness takes us to the next step: we focus on our own part in our emotional suffering through an honest (but, non-judgmental) evaluation of our own behaviors;

» We understand what happened and face our own mistake;

» Facing and taking responsibility for our own shortcoming forces us to see our humanness: we come to accept that, as an imperfect human being, we cannot be perfect;

» This understanding, acknowledgment, and acceptance empowers us to forgive ourselves for our wrongdoing;

» Self-forgiveness frees us from experiencing emotional pain and liberates us from seeing ourselves trapped—now, we see choices;

» As we evaluate our options, we realize that, even though we have no control over others, we *have* control over our own thoughts, feelings, and behaviors—we *have inner control*;

» As we see the bigger picture, we come to see other people's humanness—we see their true image (their *total self*):
   ◦ We come to accept their innate characteristics, as we do our own; and
   ◦ We understand and relate to their humanness (their flawed ways of thinking, feeling, and behaving), as we do towards our own;

» This awareness, acceptance, and compassion for other people allows us to separate their behaviors from their *person* (their *self*);

» Realizing that we have issues with their behaviors and not them as a person empowers us to reject their behaviors and not them; and, finally;

» Since we don't take things personally, we become enabled to resolve issues by expressing ourselves in a non-reactive, non-provocative, and effective communication style (i.e., *I love you but I have an issue with your behavior*). Therefore, while we still hold others accountable for their wrongdoings towards us, we don't take things personally. Taking such an impersonal view helps us forgive other people and let go of our resentment.

In conclusion, developing an understanding and forgiving mindset is an important part of our journey towards achieving total wellness: Since such a constructive mindset helps us reach a state of emotional healing, we become empowered to manage our relapses and adhere to our lifestyle changes in a more consistent manner.

12

PERCEPTIVE INNER THOUGHTS AND SELF-TALKS

This final chapter presents perceptive internal thoughts and dialogue that are driven by *a mindful, conscientious, and empathetic mindset* (i.e., a mindset that is gained through the process of personal growth and transformation). These inner thoughts and self-talks serve as a starting point on the path to emotional healing.

※ ※ ※

I realize that, while the journey of personal growth liberates me and empowers me to achieve a state of total wellness, it can initially cause emotional pain. This is because:

» As I embark on the journey of change and gain insight into my conditioned patterns of thinking, feeling, and behaving, some unresolved issues or hurtful memories from the past may resurface to the level of consciousness and create inner turmoil in me. For example,
  ◦ I may become aware of my past wrongdoings. This self-awareness may produce internal conflicts and generate such self-talks as: *I'm not good enough.*
  ◦ I may discover that I have learned many of my faulty ways of thinking, feeling, and behaving from my parents. This discovery may generate feelings of disillusionment, dismay, and sadness.
  ◦ I may become aware of my parents' shortcomings and poor parenting style that have contributed to my emotional suffering. This realization may generate intense feelings of anger and resentment.

» As I embark on my journey and discover the truth, I become aware of the wrongdoings of others towards me (particularly, those of my loved ones). This discovery may make me see myself as a victim. This perception can generate feelings of resentment, powerlessness, and helplessness.

If left unresolved, such painful thoughts and emotions may trigger a set of conditioned responses. For example, I may easily become frustrated or get defensive and snap at others; engage in denial, refuse to deal with issues, and continue to enable people; and/or, use food, alcohol, or other substances to comfort myself.

I realize that these defense mechanisms that may protect me from experiencing inner turmoil in the short term, will stop my personal growth and make me feel stuck in the long term.

Although the inner turmoil that I initially experience on my journey of change causes displeasure, I understand that it is a natural and transient part of the process. This realization helps me become more patient and supportive towards myself and resolve my inner unrest in such healthy ways as these:

» On a daily basis, I will practice relaxation techniques (e.g., meditation, deep-breathing exercises, or mindful-walking) to bring myself back to the present moment.

» I will craft, practice, and cultivate constructive and empowering self-talk scripts, such as the following:

"I believe in my inner strengths . . . I can face the truth without being judgmental or critical towards myself or other people . . .
As a mature adult, I will take responsibility for my flaws and present emotional suffering . . .
Blaming others (e.g., my parents) brings about further emotional pain . . . Perceiving myself as a victim makes me feel helpless and stuck . . . However, taking responsibility for my faulty behaviors empowers me to see choices . . ."

To forgive and gain a sense of inner calmness, refer to the inspirational scripts in the "Emotional Healing" section of *The Inner Control Is the True Control Workbook (2nd Edition)*.

*Letting go of our feelings of resentment does not mean
accepting other people's hurtful behaviors;
Nor does it mean blaming ourselves for our feelings of hurt,
anger, frustration, disgust, hatred, or jealousy . . .*

*Rather, letting go of our feelings of resentment is about
genuinely releasing such feelings so that we could emotionally
detach ourselves from those whom we resent:*

*For it is when we are emotionally free that we can think clearly,
see our choices, and lead a proactive and fulfilling life.*

*Then, in essence, to let go of our feelings of resentment is to
retake our personal power and control over our lives.*

*Let your feelings of resentment awaken and
mobilize you, not enslave you.*

*Source: A Tool for Letting Go of Resentment and Anger:
Short. Straightforward. Transformative.*

❧ ❧ ❧

Although the journey of change will empower me to form healthier relationships and enjoy more rewarding experiences, it may initially create more stress in my interactions with others. This is because I may become critical and judgmental when I begin to gain awareness and discover other people's flawed character-traits that I had not noticed before. I may even become anxious and develop a sudden urge to analyze and fix people in my immediate environment.

In such instances, I will remember that over-functioning is counterproductive and may lead to negative outcomes for everyone involved. Moreover, I will keep in mind that, as mature and capable adults, others are responsible for improving themselves and meeting their own goals. This awareness will stop me from crossing personal boundaries and fixing people.

Now, while I make a positive impact on the lives of others, I will focus on my own self-improvement and self-care.

Now, instead of expressing judgmental views or fixing people, I will *share my observations* in a supportive and empowering manner. In such a case, others will hear:

I believe in you, your abilities, and what you can accomplish.

🐦 🐦 🐦

Although I am aware that I can transform and change my lifestyle, I realize that some of my ways of thinking, feeling, and behaving that are deeply conditioned in me may be difficult to change: For example, in times of stress, some of my old habits may come back.

I will accept that returning to my old ways is a natural part of the process of change. This realization liberates me: Now, when I face setbacks, I will remember that I'm not stuck: I have choices.

> *"It is only by going down into the abyss that we recover the treasures of life. Where you stumble, there lies your treasure."* —Joseph Campbell

Now,

I will set myself up for success:

I will make realistic goals;
I will work towards progression,
not perfection; and,
I will believe in myself.

> *Please allow the Nurturing Parent within you to support and guide you on your journey.*

Accountability and Empowerment
A Four-Step Strategy for Overcoming Resentment

Accountability and Empowerment is the second book in the series of *The Inner Control Is the True Control: Making Lifestyle and Behavioral changes.*

This book empowers you to gain insight into yourself when you experience stress in your relationships:

Am I feeling annoyed? Am I feeling offended?
Or, do I feel that I've been wronged?

Do I have a tendency to compare myself with others
and experience feelings of inadequacy?

Through inspiring you to look inwardly, *Accountability and Empowerment* provides you with a tool to retake your personal power, let go of your feelings of resentment, see choices, and experience better health and quality of life.

🌸° 🌸° 🌸°

A Tool for Letting Go of Resentment and Anger
Short. Straightforward. Transformative.

A Tool for Letting Go of Resentment and Anger contains self-inquiry questions, worksheets, and inspirational words and quotes to help you let go of your feelings of resentment and prevent its downward spiral. (The diagram on the next page illustrates how holding onto resentment can negatively impact our physical and mental health).

Through asking thought provoking questions, this workbook helps you find answers when you are experiencing stress in your relationships. The inspirational words and quotes presented in this book inspire you to regain control and move onward.

This transformative *workbook* is a companion to *Accountability and Empowerment*. Although it is recommended that readers work through both books to receive the maximum benefit, you can still gain a transformative experience by exploring either one independently of the other.

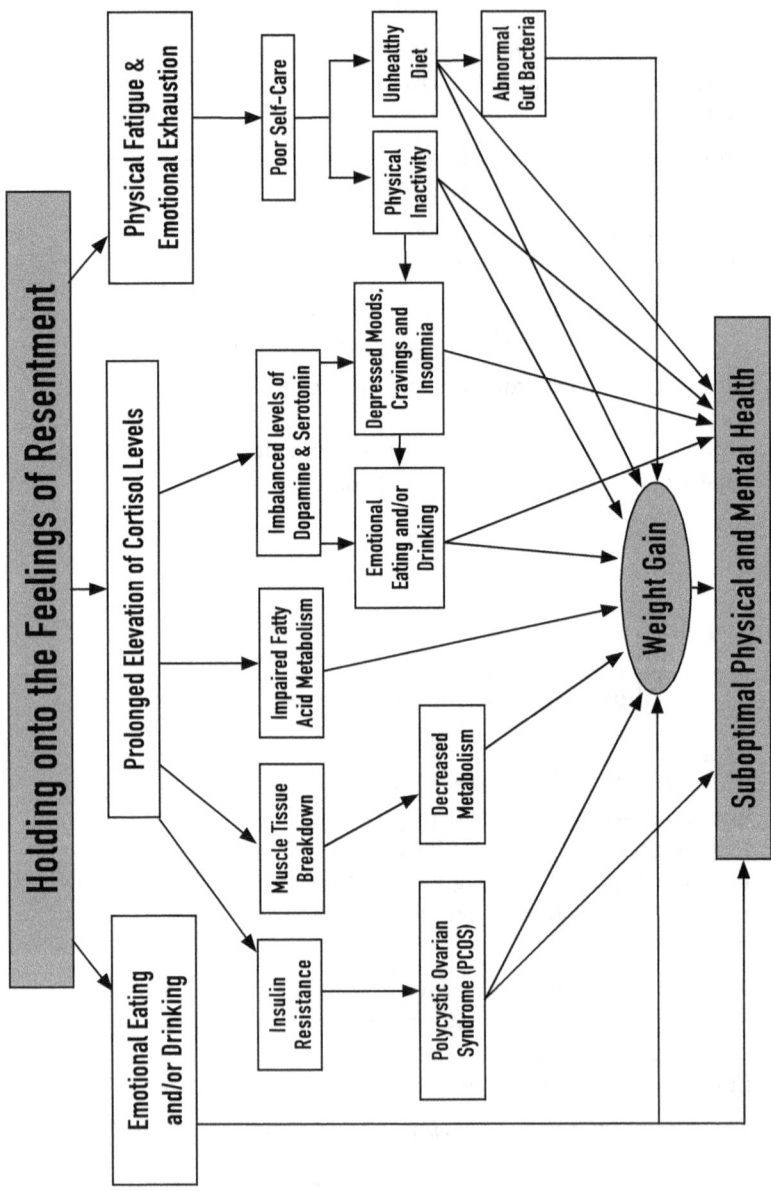

Holding onto the Feelings of Resentment

- Physical Fatigue & Emotional Exhaustion
  - Poor Self-Care
    - Unhealthy Diet
      - Abnormal Gut Bacteria
    - Physical Inactivity
- Prolonged Elevation of Cortisol Levels
  - Imbalanced levels of Dopamine & Serotonin
    - Depressed Moods, Cravings and Insomnia
    - Emotional Eating and/or Drinking
  - Impaired Fatty Acid Metabolism
  - Muscle Tissue Breakdown
    - Decreased Metabolism
  - Insulin Resistance
    - Polycystic Ovarian Syndrome (PCOS)
- Emotional Eating and/or Drinking

Weight Gain

Suboptimal Physical and Mental Health

Source: A Tool for Letting Go of Resentment and Anger: Short. Straightforward. Transformative.

References

Beck, Judith (2011). *Cognitive Behavior Therapy*. New York, NY: The Guilford Press.

Briggs, D. C. (1971). *Celebrate Your Self: Enhancing Your Own Self-Esteem*. Garden City, NY: Doubleday & Company.

Forward, Susan (1989). *Toxic Parents: Overcoming Their Hurtful Legacy and Reclaiming Your Life*. New York, NY: Bantam Books.

Germer, C., Siegel, R., & Fulton, P. (2013). *Mindfulness and Psychotherapy*. New York, NY: Guilford Press.

Gilbert, Daniel (2006). *Stumbling on Happiness*. New York, NY: Random House.

Gilbert, Roberta (1992). *Extraordinary Relationships: A New Way of Thinking About Human Interactions*. Minneapolis, MN: Chronimed Publishing.

Goleman, Daniel (1994). *Emotional Intelligence: Why It Can Matter More Than IQ*. New York, NY: Bantam Books.

Gordon, Thomas (1970). *P.E.T.: Parent Effectiveness Training*. New York, NY: Three Rivers Press.

Lister-Ford, Christine (2002). *Skills in Transactional Analysis Counseling & Psychotherapy*. Thousand Oaks, CA: Sage Publications.

Luskin, Fred (2009). *Forgive for Love: The Missing Ingredient for a Healthy and Lasting Relationship*. New York, NY: Harper Collins Publishers.

Ruiz, Don Miguel (1997). *The Four Agreements*. San Rafael, CA: Amber-Allen Publishing.

Ruiz, Don Miguel (1999). *The Mastery of Love*. San Rafael, CA: Amber-Allen Publishing.

Ruiz, Don Miguel (2004). *The Voice of Knowledge*. San Rafael, CA: Amber-Allen Publishing.

Schwartz, Barry (2004). *The Paradox of Choice: Why More is Less*. New York, NY: HarperCollins Publishers.

Sehatti, A. (2020). *Accountability and Empowerment: A Four-Step Strategy for Overcoming Resentment (2) The Inner Control Is the True Control*. Campbell, CA: NCWC/Amend-Health Press.

Sehatti, A. (2022). *The Inner Control Is the True Control Workbook: Making Lasting Lifestyle and Behavioral Changes*. 2nd Ed. Campbell, CA: NCWC/Amend-Health Press.

Seligman, Martin (2002). *Authentic Happiness*. New York, NY: Free Press.

Shannon, Joseph (2016). *Understanding Personality Disorders* [Audio-Visual DVD]. USA: Institute for Brain Potential.

Shapiro, Lawrence (1997). *How to Raise a Child with a High EQ*. New York, NY: HarperCollins Publishers.

Stone, D., Patto, B., & Heen, S. (1999). *Difficult Conversations: How to Discuss What Matters Most*. New York, NY: Penguin Books.

Tolle, Eckhart (2004). *The Power of Now: A Guide to Spiritual Enlightenment*. Vancouver, Canada: Namaste Publishing.

Walton-Moss, B., Becker, K., Kub, J., & Woodruff, K. (2013). *Substance Abuse: Commonly Abused Substances and the Addiction Process*. Brockton, MA: Western Schools.

Vander Zanden, James (1978). *Human Development*. New York, NY: Random House.

www.ingramcontent.com/pod-product-compliance
Lightning Source LLC
Chambersburg PA
CBHW072144020426
42334CB00018B/1875